"A timely message –  :art and expand your world, nd new corners."
Thea Alexander, author of *2150, A.D.*

Δ Δ Δ

"A parable for our time. Gives much to think about and use on your own path of enlightenment."
Dr. Wayne W. Dyer, author of *Gifts from Eykis*

Δ Δ Δ

"A feast of images, feelings, and ideas to nourish the soul in practical ways!"
Rev. Edie Skalitzky, Unity Minister, Seminar Leader

Δ Δ Δ

"If you have an open mind and a passion for self-discovery and love the Earth, read this book. Its message is timely — indeed crucial — at this pivotal time in our evolution."
Daniel D. Chiras, Ph.D., author of *Beyond the Fray: Reshaping America's Environmental Response*

Δ Δ Δ

"A colorful adventure of consciousness. *Owner's Manual* offers a clear and positive blueprint for successful living and a healed planet — a book with heart!"
Alan Cohen, author of *Joy is My Compass & The Dragon Doesn't Live Here Anymore*

Δ Δ Δ

Owner's Manual Quotes

Chapter 1: All wisdom, all answers are within us if we will only access them.

Fear must be conquered by releasing resistance.

Personal power and courage are best developed when we move toward the things that we love.

There are no barriers to those who release their fear.

True courage is exemplified by the peaceful — only cowards resort to acts of aggression and violence.

There will come a time when you will be greatly needed by the Living Spaceship Earth and her inhabitants.

Judgment is a lack of understanding.

Every person is your mirror. What you see in each individual is a reflection of yourself.

When you break down the walls of judgment, then you will have reached understanding.

Truth does not have to take an eternity.

Chapter 2: Truth has no effect on a closed mind.

Hold onto your dream no matter what happens. Allow nothing to prevent you from accomplishing your mission.

(More quotes on page 312.)

DO YOU HAVE
AN OWNER'S MANUAL
FOR YOUR BRAIN?

MARINA RAYE

EDITED BY CHUCK SHEPPARD

**ACTION
PRESS**™

Published by Action Press
P.O. Box 6250, Colorado Springs, Colorado 80934

Cover art by Charles Frizzell
First Edition
Although the author and publisher have exhaustively researched all sources to ensure the accuracy and completeness of the information contained in this book, we assume no responsibility for errors, inaccuracies, omissions, or any inconsistency herein. Any slights of people or organizations are due to an unintentional coincidence. Readers should use their own judgment or consult their personal physician for specific applications to their individual problems.

ISBN: 1-878010-00-X

Printed in the United States of America

TO GAIA — MAY YOU SMILE SOON

About the Author

Marina Raye has a master's degree in counseling psychology and is president of High Performance Training, Inc. Her seminars have been offered to thousands of individuals and corporations, providing practical tools to develop their *Owner's Manuals*.

Her workshops sparkle with her purposeful enthusiasm, excitement, and involvement. They are both entertaining and highly practical for today's growth-oriented individual. Her book is written in this same style — alive with energy, action, and purpose. Marina is a bright new star in a world desperately in need of light.

Marina lives in the Rocky Mountains of Colorado and has competed in the Pikes Peak Triple Crown of Running, which includes the Pikes Peak Ascent. She is a sought-after media personality and professional speaker, whose passion is the return to partnership with individuals and with the Planet Earth. She is an active change agent, helping to awaken and empower willing individuals to fulfill their higher purpose.

Her book is science faction — combining outrageous creativity with factual information — offering tools for personal and global transformation.

Chuck Sheppard, Editor
Author of *ABZ's of High Performance*

Contents

Introduction

It was late spring in the Garden of the Gods, near my home in Colorado Springs. A flaming sunset colored the sandstone rock formations a glowing orange-gold. Five deer in a grassy meadow looked up to say hello as I ran past. I was totally engrossed in my thoughts of writing the *Owner's Manual* — a book that would help people use their brain/minds in a way that supports and nurtures them and would return balance to the planet Earth.

It must be a book that will grab people's attention, steal them away from non-stop schedules, and scream, "READ ME! You owe it to yourself to READ ME!"

An *Owner's Manual* for the brain? Where do I begin?

"Stop!" commanded a Voice. I stopped. This was not a Voice to be doubted. I looked around and saw only deer, emerald green trees swaying gracefully in the breeze, a magpie whirring past — but no source of the Voice. I shrugged my shoulders and began to run when the Voice grabbed me by the throat and shouted, "Stop!"

I stopped, and in that frozen moment in time, Maya appeared, as her story — our story — unfolded like a rapid span of time and space in my consciousness. Maya's story and my life have since become so closely interwoven that I sometimes forget who is who in this fascinating discovery called an *Owner's Manual*.

The premise of this book is that wisdom is a process of remembering, that the answers to our personal and planetary healing are encoded within each individual.

The *Owner's Manual* provides tools to make your brain "user friendly" — preparing you to meet the challenges of the 21st Century, today.

One word of caution: This book is not for everyone — only for those who deserve it. Are you ready to remember your true self? Then you deserve your *Owner's Manual.* Are you on a path of spiritual growth, hungry for a deeper understanding of your higher purpose on this planet? Then you deserve your *Owner's Manual.* Do you wish for a more balanced life, a return to a life of partnership with your feminine and masculine energy? Then you deserve your *Owner's Manual.* Do you feel a deep love for the Planet Earth and want to join millions in the return to ecobalance? Then you deserve your *Owner's Manual,* for global change begins with you and with me.

Read this book with an open mind, once for pure enjoyment, and then again and again with a highlighter. The material in the Adventure chapters has been used in my training seminars with thousands of individuals and corporations, providing simple, practical tools that have changed many lives.

Allow Maya to guide you, at times gently, at times abruptly, to a place of deeper love and understanding — the path of the heart.

Congratulations — you deserve your *Owner's Manual.*

With Galactic love,

Marina Raye

Prologue

The Starchild

Every two thousand Earth years a starchild is born. There was much rejoicing in the crystal city of Cayeres when the ancient prophecy was fulfilled. It was the prophecy of a girl-child who would be born encoded with total Galactic wisdom and understanding, who at a future time, would receive Earthling encodings. Her mission — to bring love and understanding, balance and ecological harmony to a planet in grave peril.

Δ Δ Δ

The metal wings of Maya's spacebird fluttered noiselessly, a burst of flames escaping from the starship's belly. Then it smoothed to a slow-motion glide, dropping one thousand feet to a perfect landing. Maya opened the skyroof, pushed the exit lever, and with a graceful leap, landed twenty feet from her ship. She removed the clasp from her flowing, blond hair and began her run to the city. Although she could have easily transported herself in an instant, she preferred to let her long legs take her to Cayeres.

The city appeared in the distance, iridescent in the silvery shadows of a double moon. Cayeres, the ceremonial city of Maya's ancestors, was abandoned now, except for Cyruse, the white wolf.

Maya ran toward the city with the sure-footed motion of one who was totally confident and acquainted with her surroundings. Suddenly, a form of purest white floated beside her, running in perfect cadence with her strides, sharing the joy of abandonment to movement, energy, and silent communication.

As Maya and her companion entered the city of towering crystals, she heard once again the perfection, the fluidity of the tones, sounding, reverberating — the five spirit tones she had chosen as a child.

△ △ △

"You are The Chosen One, Maya," her grandmother had said. "You must select wisely, for each tone contains a gift which you will share with many. Your intuition will guide you to the perfect tones."

The child Maya had looked with awe at the crystal gallery, assorted tones sounding a jangled symphony as she moved through the gallery with excited anticipation.

"Approach each crystal slowly," her grandmother had instructed. "Stand before it and wait until there is absolute silence. Then, let your voice sound a note of your own and wait again. You will know when the right tones find you because they will mirror back to you the purest reflection of your spirit."

Power, Love, Healing, Wisdom, and Understanding were the gifts the child Maya had chosen for her spirit tones. Now she was returning on her solo space voyage from Chichen Itza, to run again through the crystal paths with her friend and companion, Cyruse, and to re-experience the color, the sound, and the feeling of each of her spirit tones.

Maya and Cyruse approached the central crystal gallery, losing themselves in a labyrinth of light and sound, Maya's five tones resounding louder and louder. Then, as suddenly as the tones had begun, they ceased, and Maya turned to look lovingly into the ice-silver eyes of Cyruse. The white wolf knowingly returned her gaze.

Cyruse had come to her as a tiny wolf pup on the day of her spirit tone ceremony, running out of the forest toward the child Maya, knowing that they were destined to be together. They had formed an immediate bond of kinship and protection and had spent many days, running through the paths of the crystal city and the nearby forest.

The white wolf had remained in Cayeres when

Maya's people had returned to Chichen Itza to complete the mission of building their colonies on the foreign planet. And yet, they were never far apart in spirit. Together now, they sat in the crystalline silence as Maya prepared to enter her Dreamtime to re-experience her spirit tones and their gifts.

Δ Δ Δ

A deep blue mist began to fill one of the passageways, drawing Maya into its opening, which shrank to a low, narrow tunnel, barely large enough for her to enter. She heard a low humming of her Power tone, resonating, filling her with its essence. Moving through the tunnel, she found herself in an open passage, the blue mist deepening into clouds of color. Broken by the rumble of thunder, the humming intensified to rise above the storm. Lightning flashed through the blue fog, as a voice echoed, "Power flows from love and acceptance. There is no fear."

Misty blue-green depths of sound led Maya to the second crystal passage. The tone of Love enveloped her as the ancient voice of the gentle whale spirit called, "Come with me, and I will keep our dream as I keep the Earth."

Maya's voice rose in a mirroring cry, "Yes, I will remember our dream — together we are love!"

The third passage led Maya to a waterfall — rippling, flowing, sounding the fluid tone of Healing. Rose-shaded light behind the sound drew her through an open doorway, leading to a glowing river, a river of jewels and crystals. A musical voice intoned, "Healing is experienced in the return to balance and harmony."

Purest spirit tone, echoing through the fourth passageway, led her higher and higher, above the tallest crystal, to a mountain of purple light. Cyruse at her side, Maya followed the tone of Wisdom, drawn into the depths of sound that whispered, "All wisdom — all knowledge is accessed by remembering."

The tone of Understanding remained, drawing her to its golden passage. There she saw the image of a child's face cloaked in innocence, aging rapidly into an ancient woman, who urged, "Understanding comes from choosing the path of the heart."

Maya felt herself being lifted through a chorus of a thousand voices, blending five purest spirit tones in celestial harmony.

△ △ △

She opened her eyes and held Cyruse in an embrace as strong and tender as the eternal bond connecting them. "Until our next adventure, beloved spirit sister," Maya whispered.

And so began the mission that would fulfill her destiny and change the course of history for the Earthlings.

PART ONE

PREPARATION FOR THE 21ST CENTURY

Chapter 1

Maya – The Perfect One

△ △ △ Chichen Itza, Yucatan, Mexico, 875 A.D. △ △ △

Maya entered the newly-completed pyramid. It was a great honor to be the first selected to experience this unique, technologically-advanced structure, the Pyramid of Past and Future Reality. Every aspect of the pyramid was engineered to enhance the Dreamtime.

As was the custom, Maya had been taught from birth into her present time-space to honor dream-state awareness. She was highly advanced in pre-programmed mind travel and unequaled in post-Dreamtime recall.

Carlos, her brother, had suggested the Dreamtime project shortly after she had received the invitation from the Galactic Council to undertake the mission of time-space travel into the 21st Century. She remembered Carlos saying, "They chose you because you are the most balanced person in our highly evolved culture. You are courageous, powerful, and action-oriented. At the same time you are the epitome of feminine energy — loving, nurturing, and intuitive — which makes you The Perfect One for this mission."

Maya felt a mixture of pride and fear — a fear that she had not experienced since childhood. She must release this emotion immediately, or be honor bound to disqualify herself from Mission *Owner's Manual*.

The pyramid door closed behind her, sealing her in absolute silence. Using an illumination rod, she found her way to the Chamber of Power. She was aware that the next few hours or days would determine her future and the future of the 21st Century.

The Dreamtime pre-programming must be perfect. *What issues must I face? Fear? Yes. Personal power? Yes. I must also access total understanding — an understanding of how to transmit our advanced brain technology to the insatiably hungry minds of 21st Century Earthlings. This will be the ultimate test of Mission Owner's Manual.*

Maya entered the circular pool filled with tiny, feathery-soft balls the size of her thumbnail. Suddenly, she was immersed in total darkness. Gravity ceased to exist as she floated in a weightless state.

She felt herself being drawn into a whirlwind of light and color. She heard the sound of five tones, at first faintly, then increasing in volume. It was the sound of absolute harmony and perfection that transported her into a different space and time.

Δ Δ Δ

She was eight years old. Carlos was swimming ahead of her in the aqua-clear lake near their home. Although dark rainclouds moved like silent ships across the azure sky, the temperature remained suffocatingly hot. Carlos, an excellent swimmer for a ten-year-old, headed toward the large outcropping of rocks in the center of the lake. She had watched him swim to it many times but had never dared to follow him until now.

Mother and Father will be proud of me, Maya thought. Carlos is swimming faster and faster, far ahead of me now. I am getting tired. My arms are so heavy. My legs will barely move.

"Help! Carlos! Help me, Carlos! Carlos!" He cannot hear me. "Carlos ... Carlos ..." Maya slipped beneath the water, her lungs starving for air, her mind fighting the fear of death. Fear! Fear! Fear! Carlos so close but so useless to me now.

Mother's voice — I can hear Mother's voice. "Relax — do not fight forces beyond your understanding. Release your resistance." Maya quickly relaxed and floated to the surface, thinking, Float! Relax! Float! Float! Float! Rest! Catch your breath. Now swim to the rocks....

"Maya, are you all right?"

"Yes, my brother. I am now. Fear must be conquered by releasing resistance."

"What are you talking about?"

"Never mind, Carlos. It is so beautiful here. I shall come back often." The scene faded — first into blue, then green, rose, blurring into violet, and gold.

Δ Δ Δ

"Maya."

"Yes, Mother."

"It is time for you to celebrate becoming a woman. You know our customs. How do you choose to enter the adult world?"

"I have given this much thought, Mother. I will run from our home to the ocean and return within three days, taking along no food or water."

"This is a major challenge. Many of our youth have selected lesser challenges without dishonor. Why have you chosen this test, Maya?"

"Because I love the ocean, and I love my home. Personal power and courage are best developed when we move toward the things that we love. It will be an adequate test of my spiritual, mental, and physical preparedness."

"Then go, my child, and return to us as a woman — a woman who will never doubt her power and courage."

Before beginning her journey into adulthood, Maya knew she must ready herself mentally and spiritually. Quieting her thoughts and attuning to her inner harmony, she focused her mind on the test which lay ahead. She mentally rehearsed until every step of the journey was fully encoded. She saw herself reaching her destination, felt her triumphant return, and heard the congratulations of her family and friends. Confident that she was fully prepared, Maya bid farewell to her parents and Carlos and began the journey with passion and a sense of urgency.

The rain-soaked jungle welcomed her, beckoning her down the shaded path. She ran beneath thick, ropy vines and branches, intertwined in a ceiling of green, splashed with sunlight. Lush, jungle blossoms reached out to caress her with their delicate petals, filling the air with a heavy fragrance.

A gentle wind joined Maya and became her companion. As she lost herself in the journey toward the ocean and her destiny, she sensed that the Earth and the sky were her allies in this passionate quest. Her strength increased as she glided over the path in a euphoric state, while her mind seemed to detach from her body. A heightened awareness of the wind, the sun, the Earth, and the sky, reminded Maya of the total harmony she experienced with all of nature.

A painted sunset of burnt orange and indigo filled the darkening sky, offering her time for refreshment and contemplation. She ate a papaya which volunteered itself from its beautiful parent tree, then reviewed the day's experiences, storing them in her memory. After pre-programming her mind, she curled beneath the protective branches of a nearby sapodilla tree and soon drifted into her Dreamtime....

Δ Δ Δ

Closer and closer the giant jungle cat crept, until his emerald eyes met Maya's startled gaze.

I must not move. I must show no fear, she thought. Mother taught me that all animals can sense my thoughts and will only attack a frightened victim. Maya began to breathe deeply, sending thoughts of love and acceptance to the jaguar, now close enough for her to see his teeth and powerful muscles. She felt his hot breath on her face, as the animal released a roar that shook the ground beneath her, yet she still did not move.

Abruptly, the giant cat lay down beside her, making a loud, purring sound. Maya sensed that the jaguar was inviting her into his world. "May I ride on your back?" she asked.

His eyes acquiesced, and she leaped gracefully onto the back of the powerful animal. The next moment they were off on a moonlit ride through a mystical jungle.

The semi-darkness enveloped them, sending shadows scurrying from their path. Maya experienced the pure joy of every bounding leap through heavy underbrush which opened to a rolling meadow. Faster and faster they raced through the tall grasses, leaping over rocks and fallen trees, finally coming to a halt as the meadow gave way to jungle. The sounds of the tropical night — the singing of the locusts, the rustle of the wind — intensified as the jaguar stood majestically in the spotlight of a silver moon. Maya slid from his back and turned to face the giant cat as his thoughts entered her understanding.

"I salute you, Maya. Your people speak of me as the

Warrior because I have no fear. There are no barriers to those who release their fear. Take the gift of my courage with you on the journey through time which is your destiny. You will lead many to understand that true courage is exemplified by the peaceful — only cowards resort to acts of aggression and violence."

Δ Δ Δ

Maya awoke when the first rays of gold-orange sunlight announced the new day. After contemplating the jaguar's gift and storing her Dreamtime, she sat quietly under the sapodilla tree, aligning herself with her higher purpose and accessing a state of perfect harmony. Then she jumped up, energized and ready to continue her journey. She began her run, moving without conscious effort over the sandy path.

As the sun traveled slowly off the horizon, she could sense that she was getting close to her destination. She breathed deeply of the salty air. And then she heard it — at first faintly, and soon louder and louder — that endless, pounding, roar of the surf. I am almost there, she thought. I feel as though I am flying!

Through the tall sea grasses she caught her first glimpse of the ocean and began running even faster. She reached the shore, panting, and paused to drink in the beauty of the morning sun dancing across the sparkling waves. Next she gave thanks to the water spirits and dove into an aqua wave, which carried her high on its crest before hurling her toward the shore.

Exhilarated, Maya lay on the wet sand, filling her senses with the perfection of the moment, her bare skin delighting in the warmth of the sun after the coolness of the water. There was time for another swim before her return journey.

Swimming beyond the surf, she experienced a deep calm. She felt a bond with the ocean — a sense of oneness with this great body of water. Suddenly her reverie was interrupted by an explosion of sound and movement. All around her the water began to churn with swirling, rolling waves, and Maya intuitively sensed the presence of a strong, spiritual energy nearby.

She centered herself and treaded water, preparing for the presence that she sensed observing her. Suddenly, out of the frothing water, almost close enough to touch, appeared a huge eye and the head of a ... a ... it could not be — yet it must be — a whale!

She had heard many legends about the ancient creatures referred to as the Keepers of the Earth. Maya felt herself drawn into the depths of the eye that met her gaze. The next moment she was overcome by love flooding her entire being. This enormous creature was communicating Galactic love to her, and she returned her essence of pure love and acceptance.

Gently back and forth the silent communications flowed. "You are love in its purest form, Maya. You are recognized by our species as an advanced being who has been called to greatness. We are your allies in the mission you will undertake. We serve as guardians of the Earth, protecting the delicate harmony that keeps all life forms in balance. There will come a time when you will be greatly needed by the Living Spaceship Earth and her inhabitants. Humankind will, out of ignorance and forgetfulness, cause much damage to this beautiful planet. After many years of sleep, there will be a Great Awakening among humans, and you will be the One who will join us in creating a new world of peace, harmony, and ecological balance."

Maya closed her eyes to fully receive the message from the mammoth creature. When she refocused her gaze, the whale was gone, and she was drawn slowly back to shore. She sat in the shade of a small sea fern, releasing herself to the crystalline silence of pure awareness.

It was mid-afternoon when Maya was jolted back to the present reality by a lone seagull who communicated, "Go now, gentle Sister. There is much to be done."

Δ Δ Δ

The village appeared strangely quiet as Maya approached her home, just prior to sunset on the third day of her journey. She was disappointed. Where were Carlos, her mother, and father?

With the sound of singing, accompanied by drums, her family and friends suddenly appeared from behind rocks and trees. The celebration lasted for hours. It was Maya's day! Courage and power were hers, for she had earned them through understanding, and — more important — through action. As was the custom, she revealed to no one the details of her journey into maturity.

The vision faded again in an arc of brilliant colors....

Δ Δ Δ

"Maya, what steps must I take to develop my *Owner's Manual?*"

Maya wondered how many times she had been asked that question at the Advanced Awareness Center where she had instructed for over ten Earth years. All of her trainees had been successful in developing their *Owner's Manuals*. Many had left the Earth plane and were now serving as Galactic Agents.

Awareness and understanding — that is what must be stressed. We must be aware of the total communications process and understand much more than just the spoken word. How do we access information that is stored in our brain? How do we know when we have achieved the transmission of our thoughts into another's information system? The answers are simple, yet must be taught again and again to each new learner.

Why must individuals develop a personal *Owner's Manual?* Because each brain/mind is uniquely different and individually encoded with its higher purpose. The

Owner's Manual provides tools that interpret the encodings, allowing individuals to take ownership of their lives and fulfill their higher purpose.

Maya's image of the Advanced Awareness Center was beginning to fade, when suddenly the soft, Galactic music increased in volume, and the radiant face of Josh came bursting through an arc of spectral colors. Josh was Maya's most brilliant learner, who had often challenged her understanding of pragmatic brain technology. There was only one flaw that kept him from advancing as rapidly as they both would have liked. That flaw was his frequent judgment of his fellow learners.

Josh approached her with no hesitancy. "Maya, I have distinguished myself in your training classes. Although I have never failed to assimilate all information into my personal *Owner's Manual,* I realize that my perfection's quest has been delayed due to my 'flaw,' as you call it. I mean no harm when I am judgmental. To me, it is simply comparison. What must I do to transcend this difficulty?"

"Josh, you are beautiful mentally and physically, and your interest in perfection is a commendable trait. The answer to your question is simple, as are all answers to complex problems. Judgment is a lack of understanding. I repeat, judgment is a lack of understanding. If you see someone who appears to have an annoying character flaw, then imagine yourself being that person and live with the flaw until you understand that you and they are the same. Every person is your mirror. What you see in each individual is a reflection of yourself. When you break down the walls of judgment, then you will have reached understanding.

"My recommendation for your most rapid growth," continued Maya, "is for you to choose to occupy a body that has no physical beauty, while retaining your brilliant mind." Moments later, the image of Josh shrank to that of a physically grotesque being, then disappeared into a rainbow of color.

Δ Δ Δ

Harmonic tones pulsating through her awareness, Maya floated gently to the top of the magic pool. The glow of the illumination rod became visible as she returned to conscious awareness. She reviewed and stored her Dreamtime for future access.

She stepped out of the pool, moving quickly toward the exit. Carlos greeted her outside the door of the Pyramid of Past and Future Reality. "You appear transformed, my sister."

"Yes. All wisdom, all answers are within us if we will only access them. The Pyramid is a transformational tool in helping us to remember our inner wisdom. How long was I inside?"

"Two hours!"

"You are not serious. Two hours?"

"Yes. Truth does not have to take an eternity."

"Carlos, I am ready to accept my mission without fear — with power, courage, awareness, and understanding. When do we meet with the Galactic Council?"

"It is scheduled on the day of the Equinox. I am honored to be your brother, Maya. You are the future!"

Chapter 2

You Are The Future

Maya closed her eyes, creating a vision of what it would be like to be on the Living Spaceship Earth in the 21st Century. Feelings of sorrow and pain engulfed her as images flashed onto her mental screen.

"I see many people looking lost and confused — sending out a myriad of mixed signals. It is unfortunate to see such magnificent equipment as their brain/minds being ineffectively operated. Look on your screen, Carlos," she whispered, her eyes filling with tears of compassion. "Most of them are not aware that their minds have predictable and controllable patterns. They are allowing their brains to run unconsciously, while they spend most of their time preoccupied with the past or the future, failing to cherish the present moment."

"They do emit a feeling of exhaustion," replied Carlos, "as if they are trying to burn themselves up, consumed by their own powers." A lightning bolt flashed across their screens, followed by an explosion of thunder, fading out the images.

"It is time for me to go to the Advanced Awareness

Center," stated Maya. "Do you want to come with me? All the learners adore you!"

"And I them," her brother replied, "but not today. I must stay in the Observatory to make our final chrono-metric calculations. You are certain about your decision, are you not? The Galactic Council meets on the day of the Equinox, and Mission *Owner's Manual* must be encoded soon if we are to make the transport safely."

"I perceive that this mission is my destiny, and it is an honor to have been chosen. And yet, I will miss returning to our home galaxy and our family."

"You have made the right choice. Of that I am sure, my sister," Carlos replied gently. "The Earth desperate-ly needs your perfect balance of feminine and masculine energy. The 21st Century is an age of acceptance and nurturing of the intuitive spirit — called 'right-brain enhancement.' The Earthlings are ready to accept your guidance. In addition, your power and courage will inspire many to action. And our knowledge of time-space travel will make it reasonably safe for you to transport to the future."

"What do you mean, 'reasonably safe?'"

"You will be our first transport with complete Galactic and Earthling encodings. There are some unknowns involved."

"I need to be aware of these unknowns, so that I may prepare myself."

"Well spoken, Maya. Here are my concerns. How well will you acclimate as an Earthling? You may have difficulty retaining Dreamtime awareness, and you may become trapped in lower astral planes if you do not remain in harmony with your Galactic frequency."

"There is something else. What is it?"

"I am concerned as to how soon you will be able to access all your Galactic memories. If you do so too quickly, the mission will have to be aborted because your full Galactic powers would overwhelm the Earthlings. You might be held in awe, perhaps feared by some, or even held captive physically."

"I understand, Carlos. I will prepare myself through brain/mind programming and through attunement to my higher purpose. Then I will anchor the programming to my harmonic frequency so that I will be able to access my Galactic resources at the perfect time."

Δ Δ Δ

Later that evening, Maya entered the cool recesses of the Dream Temple. It was here that she was able to commune with her mother and father who had already returned to their Galactic home of Mayata. She sipped the sweet nectar brought to her by the white-robed priestess, Xtaban. "Are you going to contact your parents in Mayata again?"

"Yes, and this may be my last conscious communication with them for some time."

"Just remember to be attuned to the harmonic frequency that will guide your consciousness to Mayata," Xtaban suggested.

Moments later Maya sensed subtle currents drawing her into a vast emptiness. She began to resonate with five tones of purest harmony as a sudden shift in her energy field opened her inner screen to the sight of her Galactic homeland and the parents she loved and respected.

"Maya," her father began, "we miss your presence. We are honored that you have been chosen to represent our entire Galactic evolution. Yours is the most important mission Mayata has ever undertaken. You will touch billions of lives and help to save the Earthlings from self-destruction."

"It will soon be time for you to begin your journey," her mother stated. "The 21st Century needs your harmony. Your mission is to lead the way for the Earthlings of the future to remember their true selves and to return their planet to balance and harmony. These beings have turned life into a struggle, although it is not intended to be difficult to live a happy and fulfilling existence. The Earthlings are equipped with advanced brain/mind technology of which few are aware. They must learn to operate their magnificent brains at a higher level and take ownership of their lives, or they will destroy themselves and their beautiful Living Spaceship Earth. You will guide them, Maya, by helping them to discover the path that will lead them back to themselves."

"I honor your wisdom and understanding, Mother. This is the mission I have been preparing for since the beginning of time. For the Earthlings, their transformation will seem to be a step backwards into the future.

"Father, you appear troubled about something. What is it?"

"Maya, I would be less than truthful if I did not relate to you the contents of a recent dream. It was the most unusual dream that I have ever experienced. It left me feeling a strange foreboding, but I am sure that it was ..."

"Father, please, what happened?"

"It was a rapid view of the history of the Earthling civilization. Many great beings from Socrates to the Kennedy brothers are killed by their own society. Think about it — Socrates, John the Baptist, Jesus, Joan of Ark, Lincoln, Gandhi, King, and many more."

"You are saying that my life will be in danger?"

"Yes, constantly. Your face was the last image in this nightmare of a dream."

"Was I being killed?"

"No. You appeared radiantly healthy and happy. Perhaps the dream was telling us that the development of *Owner's Manuals* will forever stop the dramatic assassination of the most enlightened beings. But maybe ... maybe it was warning us that you will be next. Simply be aware of non-receptive individuals. Remember two points — truth has no effect on a closed mind, and it always takes less effort to kill an idea than it does to implement it."

"Father, I accept your warning in the loving spirit in which it is given. I am willing to give my life for only one cause — that cause is Mission *Owner's Manual* — which will create more happiness and peace of mind than any discovery in the history of humankind."

Her mother added a solemn reminder. "Maya, Maya, maintain your awareness. Hold onto your dream no matter what happens. Allow nothing to prevent you from accomplishing your mission — to guide with love and understanding."

"Please do not be overly concerned about my well-being. I feel totally protected on Mission *Owner's Manual,* but I gladly accept your harmony and Galactic guidance. I love you both. Thank you for being my soul-parents."

Both parents smiled proudly at Maya and then looked at each other, confirming their own love. They gradually faded from her inner screen in a cloud of golden light.

Maya returned to full consciousness, at peace with her ultimate challenge, and ready to meet with the Galactic Council. She was beginning to feel the excitement of her adventure into the unknown. The apprehension of leaving her family was gone, replaced with a passion to begin her journey. Her path would contain adventure, as well as challenges, and perhaps even danger, but she was ready for what lay ahead. She must handle Mission *Owner's Manual* without a single flaw. She also remembered her father's warning about how

Earthling societies had dealt with "perfect" beings....

Δ Δ Δ

Maya entered the stately chambers of the Galactic Council. The Council Leader, High Priestess Tuluma, began speaking immediately. "Welcome, Maya. We are pleased that you have chosen to accept this mission. As an Earthling, your consciousness of your powers will be severely limited. It is for your safety that your Earthly contact with us can only take place in your Dreamtime. You will remember your powers gradually, just as the Earthlings must. But you will not be alone. There are those on the Living Spaceship Earth with heightened awareness who are already expecting you. In addition, you will be under the constant protection of our Galactic Agents."

Maya listened intently to the Council Leader who continued, "You will be going to a country called the United States of America. This country has been a leader in the field which the Earthlings call high technology. The people have an openness and acceptance of concepts and ideologies associated with personal freedom. Yet their ideals, their hopes and dreams have become clouded by a mechanistic society dedicated to materialism. Government bureaucracies, military extremism, religious bigotry, and personal greed have created strong controlling groups. These groups are of the mindset that war can protect economic interests and are quick to engage in military confrontation, rather than peaceful resolution of conflicts.

"There is much fear, particularly of illness, called disease, which reflects a lack of ease that the Earthlings have with themselves and their surroundings. In addition, rather than nurturing their Living Spaceship Earth, the Earthlings exhibit negligence and abuse caused by an attitude of superiority over all other planetary life forms.

"The Earthlings are on a collision course with a grim destiny. Unless global changes are made, their host planet is in grave danger of being destroyed. Lack of harmony with nature has brought about a critical level of what is called pollution. Their 'high technology' has caused massive amounts of toxic wastes to be released into the atmosphere of their fragile planet. They have poisoned their oceans and their fresh water supplies. Even the air they breathe and the food they eat is contaminated. Now that it is almost too late, they are frantically searching for answers — answers that the *Owner's Manual* will help them to access from within themselves.

"Everything has been arranged for your adaptation — your home, your personal belongings, your credentials — all you will need to function as a member of the Earthlings' society.

"You will speak the language flawlessly. You will be encoded with all the memories appropriate to your time and place. Your education will be that of a writer and what is called a neuro-linguistic psychologist. I perceive that you have questions."

"Yes. How long will I remain in the 21st Century? How will I know when my mission is fully accomplished? Will I return to Chichen Itza or Mayata?"

"You will return when your original mission is completed. The concept of an *Owner's Manual* for the brain will be embraced with few exceptions. To stay longer than necessary would only cause some Earthlings to design a religious-type following for you. Your outcome is to be an active change agent by helping to awaken and empower willing individuals to fulfill their higher purpose. The *Owner's Manual* will provide them with the tools to successfully accomplish that higher purpose.

"At times you will sense that individuals are becoming dependent on you or worshiping you rather than looking within themselves for their answers. Encourage them to internalize your message — to realize that they must be their own guru. You are simply the catalyst for them to develop their *Owner's Manuals.*

"You will return to Mayata. There will be other missions to other futures, and you will be our best prepared Galactic Agent for those missions. Remember, you are a partner with the Earthlings, Maya, the example of how life will be for them when they choose to access their *Owner's Manuals.*"

"Where will Carlos be during my time-space travel?"

"Our work on the Earth plane is almost completed for now, and Carlos will return to Mayata with the majority of us. He will be as close as your Dreamtime, however.

"After you bid your farewells, go to the Pyramid of Past and Future Reality, where Carlos will facilitate your transport. Your success will be a mirror of our Galactic evolution. Please accept our love and harmony."

Δ Δ Δ

Maya left the Galactic Council meeting with a burning intensity to begin her mission. This was the day of the Equinox, the time of transformation, and the time for her rebirthing into the 21st Century — the most critical period in the history of the Living Spaceship Earth. Her anticipation expressed itself as she greeted Carlos. "This is the day, at last!"

"Yes, my sister. Are you afraid?"

"No. I have walked through my fears, and they are behind me. There is time, my brother, for us to revisit some childhood memories."

"Yes, Maya. I would enjoy that."

Arm in arm, they left the temple and walked toward the Observatory. When they reached the stone structure, they seated themselves in the exact position for the moment when the sun would pass the circular columns and illuminate the entire room. Bathed in brilliant, golden light, they entered an altered state of consciousness, traveling through time and space to their memories....

Δ Δ Δ

"Look, Maya. There it is. Shall we swim to the outcropping of rocks in our lake?"

"Of course, Carlos." Together they reached the giant rocks, pulling themselves up onto the smooth surface to bask in the sunlight.

"It was here that I conquered fear. I almost drowned the first day I swam out to these rocks," Maya stated. "I never told you that."

"I knew that something had occurred because you appeared transformed. I will always remember what you said — 'fear must be conquered by releasing resistance.'"

"I learned to release my fear, and in that release, I found power — remembered power."

"My sister, your power is a gift that you will share with many."

"I am so happy at this moment that if the mission did not succeed, and if something did not work properly, that ..."

"What are you saying? Everything is in readiness. I have performed our calculations over and over, and there will be no problems."

"I am saying that if I should never appear in bodily form in any dimension again, that at this moment, my life is complete, so full of joy and peace. I want you to know that before I begin my journey."

"And well I understand, Maya, for I feel the same. I release my fear for your future, because I know that your spirit is eternal. Your essence will live forever."

"Let us travel to my favorite place now." Together

they moved forward on the wind, floating through time and space. Faster and faster they traveled, until they reached the shore of that great body of water that Maya considered her friend.

In the sparkling glow of the afternoon light they swam side by side, strong and powerful, diving into the surf, reappearing, only to seize the next exploding wave. After their swim, they walked along the shore, warm sand caressing their bare feet, the ocean breeze moving lightly across their bodies. The pounding of the surf harmonized with the cry of the seagulls, sounding a timeless melody.

As the brilliant sun began to melt into the blue of the water, they were drawn to the highest point overlooking the ocean. "Carlos, according to the legends, this land is sacred, and it is critical that we come to this high place to honor the wisdom of the ancients. Mission *Owner's Manual* will help to awaken humankind to their responsibility to honor all life, especially the life of the Living Spaceship Earth."

Moving higher and higher, they came to a rock formation that led to sheer, jagged cliffs overlooking the entire peninsula. "Your journey into the future is a sacred one, Maya. Although we will not be able to communicate on a conscious level, remember that I am as close as your Dreamtime. I will be attuned to your harmonic frequency so that we can communicate at the appropriate times."

Sister and brother, mirror images of one another, looked long into each other's souls, sharing the greatest of visions. Aligning their energies, they sat on the rocks in silence....

Maya's eyes opened slowly, as she sensed a presence nearby. Next to her foot was a magical creature — bright yellow, with burnt orange and black stripes. Its eyes met hers with a look of respect and recognition.

There was no fear from either, simply total acceptance. The next moment it was gone.

Maya had been taught by her mother to understand the significance of encounters such as this. She exclaimed to Carlos, "Did you see it?"

"See what?"

"The symbol — the coral snake."

"Where?"

"It was right beside me. It represents transformation and symbolizes my acceptance into the future. Carlos, I am ready. We must go now."

Δ Δ Δ

Together they entered the Pyramid of Past and Future Reality. The darkness blanketed Maya's momentary anxiety as Carlos gently guided her into a deep theta state of consciousness. Her next reality would be the 21st Century.

A sharp pain convulsed her body as she began the process of birthing this new reality. Rather than resisting the pain, she breathed deeply, releasing herself to it and to Mission *Owner's Manual*. This pain would not have to be re-experienced. Maya's acceptance of her mission represented the return to balance and harmony for the Earthlings and the Living Spaceship Earth.

Just before she released consciousness, the sound of her spirit tones flowed into her awareness. The five tones were now her magic carpet to the 21st Century.

PART TWO

MISSION
OWNER'S MANUAL

Chapter 3

The First Step into the 21st Century

"**I** know this is going to work — we've just got to find her!" Rich Land slammed down the receiver and turned to his assistant. "The show starts in two weeks, and we still haven't found the right host! Let's go back over the candidates again to see if we've overlooked someone."

"Here's one — degree in media communications, anchor for our affiliate in L.A. — all the right stuff," responded his assistant.

"Nope, qualifications are too predictable. We've got a dozen like her. I want someone different. This is no ordinary talk show. Since our theme is adventures in human potential and personal power, someone with straight news experience just won't work because, chances are, they would be far too left-brained. This calls for someone special — highly creative, energetic, powerful, even controversial. I know she's out there somewhere, looking for us as a platform for change.

"Wait a minute! We did a story on a neuroscientist

at Stanford, the one who's been involved with all the brain/mind research. Her name is Dr. Windemere — Helen, I think. See if you can find her phone number. I have an idea...."

Δ Δ Δ

Maya opened her eyes slowly, blinking in the morning sunlight that flooded the room. For a few moments, her mind felt totally empty.

Who am I? Where am I? She looked around the vaguely familiar room, adjusting to the surroundings. This is my room. These are my things, but why do I feel as though I have been on a long journey?

She completed a series of graceful centering and brain integration movements. Then she glanced at an appointment book lying open on the dresser. Lunch at the Whole Earth Cafe with Dr. Helen Windemere. Hm ... that is today. Now I remember. My lunch appointment is to discuss my research on developing an *Owner's Manual* for the brain with the head of the brain/mind research program at Stanford University. This will be a good contact for me. She will know a way to make this information available to all people.

Maya turned on the television in time to catch the day's top news stories: "Student rioting, new ecological illness, accidents, murders, giant oil spill, toxic air ..."

When is the media going to feature some good news? And when are people going to learn that life does not have to be a struggle? We have to remember how to use our *Owner's Manuals* for change to occur. Where is the leadership we need? There seems to be a growing concern, but not enough positive action that makes a difference.

She stepped out on the deck, catching her breath at the mountain glory surrounding her. An overnight rain had left an icing of snow on the mountain top, half-hidden in feathery clouds. The gold-yellow splashes of early fall accentuated the rugged expanse of foothills. A gentle breeze stirred the trees into a flowing dance. The birds, squirrels, even a rabbit munching on late-blooming wildflowers in the back yard — all were involved in the rhythm of life — a natural harmony and balance.

All of nature fulfills its purpose and does so flawlessly — except human beings, who are the only ones to fight wars, cause ecodisasters, and accept disharmony and imbalance. Why do people turn their lives into such an intense struggle, choosing fear over love, resistance over acceptance, and attitude without action? If only they had an *Owner's Manual* for their brains, then they would take ownership of their lives and remember how to live in balance and harmony.

Maya ended her contemplation with the knowledge that the answers she had discovered in her extensive brain/mind research were answers to questions facing many people: Why am I really here? How do I overcome years of dysfunctional programming? What actions can I take to control stress and access peace of mind? How do I break through barriers to my potential? How can I make a difference in the world? What can I do to return balance and harmony to the Planet Earth?

Δ Δ Δ

"Maya, I love the title of your research project," began Dr. Helen Windemere. "It just hasn't made any sense to me that such highly sophisticated equipment as the human brain doesn't have an accompanying *Owner's Manual*. And now you've been able to compile vital information that can make a big difference — if people will only utilize your ideas. I believe humankind is ready."

"Thank you, Helen. Your support is important to me. I am ready to make this information available to people throughout the world."

"And I have just the solution! It's no accident that I am lecturing in your city this week and that we are meeting for lunch. I received a call from my secretary before I left my hotel that a hot-shot television producer is looking for the perfect person to host an internationally syndicated talk show. When I talked to the producer, Rich Land, I discovered that this is no ordinary program. It's called 'High Performance Adventure,' and Rich wants to talk to you about hosting the show. It involves conducting live interviews with experts in the fields of brain/mind research, communications, and human potential. In addition, it's a live show, so there will be audience interaction. When I described your work to Rich, he insisted on meeting you immediately. He'll be joining us any moment. I hope you don't mind."

Maya was about to say that this was the opportunity that she had been seeking when they were interrupted by, "You've got to be her! Where have you been?"

Maya glanced up, and quickly answered, "It was not time yet." Then shaking her head slightly, "Excuse me. We have not met. My name is Maya Cristal, and you must be Rich Land."

"You mean Dr. Maya Cristal," added Rich. "I've heard rave reviews about your work. Some even say your views on personal empowerment border on the radical. I mean, what would happen to this world if everyone believed that whatever they dreamed, they could create? Poets and philosophers have espoused this theory for centuries, but no one paid much attention until now. You actually say you can help people develop a how-to manual for their brain, something you call an *Owner's Manual*. In the wrong hands this stuff could be extremely manipulative, even dangerous!"

Rich rubbed his hands together in excitement. "Viewers will love this! It will shoot our ratings sky-high, and then next season ..."

"Rich," Maya interrupted. "Although I am open to discussion of this position, I want to make myself clear.

I am not interested in Hollywood sensationalism. Hype is meaningless, while truth is vital to me. The program will be a success, but I require the highest integrity in its production and promotion."

"Good. I can see you're serious about this." Rich respected Maya's directness, and knew, more than ever, that she was the One. "Why don't I have the contracts drawn up, and we can go over them tomorrow morning around 8:30 at my office."

"I will be there. Oh, by the way, Rich, do you have an *Owner's Manual* for your brain?"

"Not yet. I was hoping you could see that I receive one."

"No, I cannot. No one can give you your *Owner's Manual*. You must do that for yourself. You will soon understand that all the information needed to operate our brains at high levels of consciousness is already encoded in our cellular memories. We must each develop an individual *Owner's Manual* for optimum effectiveness."

"I, uh ... well, I thought ... never mind. Thank you for arranging this meeting, Dr. Windemere. I'll see you tomorrow, Maya."

Δ Δ Δ

That evening Maya went to sleep totally confident that the perfect opportunity had presented itself. She visualized her first guests on the program, heard the conversations, and felt the thrill of knowing that because of the *Owner's Manual,* she would be able to influence many people to use their brain/minds in a way few had dreamed possible. The tools available would open doors to using maximum potential for highly conscious living and would create change in a world that was desperately in need of a different direction, a path that led beyond technology — the path of the heart.

Chapter 4

Dreamstalker

"**M**aya, Maya, maintain your awareness. Hold onto your dream ..." Maya awoke with a start, retaining an uneasy feeling that she could not identify. Did I hear someone calling my name? Impossible. I must have been dreaming. She drifted into a restless sleep — images of light and happiness, quickly changing into menacing shadows.

Suddenly, it seemed as though a crushing weight were pressing down on her mind. Unable to move, she tried to scream but could not utter a sound. Her mind was struggling, fighting against an unknown power that gripped her. I must rely upon my inner resources. There must be a way out, she thought.

"No, no, Maya, there is no escape. You are mine for the rest of eternity!" These statements were uttered by a hoarse, rasping voice, followed by sickening laughter. "You are lost, little one, lost between worlds. Let's see what happens to your dreams now!"

Maya gasped for air, feeling the tightening of a death grip on her mind. "Who ... who are you? What do you want?"

"You mean you don't recognize me? How ridiculous! I have been aware of you for eons of time, waiting for you to venture into my domain. My name is Dreamstalker. I have the delightful task of devouring the lovely dreams of unsuspecting souls like yours who lose their way between worlds. But our life together won't be so bad. You will see! Now come with me."

Maya felt herself being drawn downward — downward into inky blackness — spiraling further and further into the void. I must remember how to save myself … myself? Who am I? What is happening that I am losing all sense of being?

A numbness settled over her spirit, as she stopped struggling. Her tortured mind searched for answers, and finally, from a pinpoint of light that appeared in her mind, she heard the words, "Allow nothing to prevent you from accomplishing your mission — to guide with love and understanding."

"To guide with love and understanding?" Guide whom? What mission? Maya gave in to her exhaustion and stopped struggling. Then she heard it again. "Allow nothing to prevent you … your only enemy is fear, and only fear can give others the power to destroy you."

Yet another voice echoed in her memory, "Love your fear, and it will release you." Maya centered her awareness, reaching down to search the ground inside the glass dome that now surrounded her. She felt a large rock at her feet. Struggling to lift it, she hurled it against the glass that held her captive. A loud shattering sound was followed by an agonizing scream.

She whispered to the darkness around her, "Dreamstalker, there is nothing to fear. You must be starved for love and understanding — perhaps I can help."

Maya's eyes gradually focused on a slimy creature

— half man, half dragon — who slithered from behind a huge rock. Scales covered his arms, his neck, his hideous face.

"Maya, you wicked creature, what have you done? No one has ever dared to face me without fear. It is destroying me! How can you look upon me and know me for what I am — a poor, miserable, love-starved creature? You have spoiled it all, ruined my plan! Go away and leave me alone in my misery! Your power is too great for me, and I am doomed to forever steal the dreams of lesser spirits."

"Be aware, Dreamstalker, that when people develop their *Owner's Manuals,* there will be no lesser spirits."

Δ Δ Δ

Maya awoke with the words, "Allow nothing to prevent you from accomplishing your mission," echoing over and over in her mind. She felt a haunting sense of having escaped disaster, and yet she experienced no fear, only anticipation. "High Performance Adventure" would soon begin, and she was totally prepared to offer the *Owner's Manual* to the world.

Chapter 5

No Compromise

"Congratulations, Maya — to you, to me, to our *STAR* Network and its affiliates, and the millions of people who are going to love this show. Now that we have all the details ironed out, I've got a line-up of guests for you to look over."

"Thank you, Rich, but I will not be needing your list. We agreed that I would have the final say on the guests for the program."

"Come on, Maya. You can't possibly do all the leg-work yourself. It would take too much time, and besides, we have all the right connections."

"Rich, I cannot compromise on this issue."

"Okay. Okay. Who would you have on first?"

"My first guest will be P. J. White."

"Never heard of him. Who is he, some hot-shot entrepreneur or something?"

"The initials stand for Panhandler Joe. He is a professional panhandler from New York City's Bowery Street."

"He's what? A panhandler — you're joking, right?

Please say you're joking."

"No, I am not joking, Rich."

"I can't stand it! My whole career in ruins. The much-awaited talk show of the decade panned by critics and viewers alike because you want to start the show with a bum!"

Matching his intensity, Maya said sternly, "Rich, sit down, remain silent, and listen! And you absolutely must *not* visualize disaster. That is not possible. Panhandler Joe is a legend who has turned his profession into an art form. He is a well known and respected citizen of the Bowery because of his contributions to the community — particularly his work with abused children. He has written a book called *Getting in Step,* which is highly informative as well as entertaining. Our viewers will be intrigued by his story."

"I can't believe this is actually happening to me! All right, I give up. But this had better work. Who else do you have lined up?"

"You will be pleased with our second guest, Dr. Johanna Powers, a Ph.D. from Harvard and author of six books. Dr. Powers is highly respected for her research in the field of advanced communications technology."

"Well, that's more the type guest I had pictured. Maya, I can see that working with you is going to be an interesting experience. For some crazy reason I'm going to go along with you on P. J. White. Just be sure you know what you're doing."

"Rich, when people have completed their *Owner's Manuals,* they always know what they are doing."

Chapter 6

The Rapport Adventure

"**G**ood evening. Welcome to 'High Performance Adventure.' I am your guide, Maya Cristal. Tonight we embark on an adventure that will challenge you to formulate a personal Owner's Manual for your brain.

"Our purpose is to offer you a set of tools that will provide the information and stimulus to develop software for your brain. Your Owner's Manual will influence you in making positive and dramatic changes — so that you can enjoy high performance results in all areas of your life. Most important, you will gain a deeper understanding of yourself and your higher purpose. This will aid in your development of more positive relationships with others and with our host planet, the Living Spaceship Earth.

"All of the guests on 'High Performance Adventure' will bring us their unique insight and experience, along with a vital segment of information for your Owner's Manual.

"Our first guest has published a book entitled **Getting in Step**, which tells about his learning experiences *in an unusual profession — panhandling. Please welcome Panhandler Joe White!"*

"Yo, Maya. What a trip to be on your show!"

"Thank you, Joe. It is a pleasure to have you as our first guest. Please share your background with us."

"Well, I grew up in Brooklyn, ya know, all the usual stuff. I went off to college, got a B.A. from Pepperidge U. Then I went back to my old neighborhood, tried a couple of different jobs, even tried workin' for the family business before I eventually settled into what I'm doin' now."

"And you have been quite successful."

"Well, I've turned a few bucks, ya know."

"Tell us about your book."

"*Getting in Step* is all about how I learned to be the best at what I do. I mean, why bother, if you can't be the best, right? It's got lots of stories — some funny, some sad, some sorta scary."

"How do you get in step with people, Joe?"

"Well, the down-and-outers, the winoes — you know the type — some of them act blind or lame, somethin' pitiful like that. And they just sit on the street with their tin cups and beg. Now, that's got no class, ya know. When I started my career, I noticed the really successful guys didn't wait for people to feel sorry for them. They'd walk alongside a likely target, pacin' their manner of walkin', body posture, even their breathin'. Then they'd wait for the right moment, look the person in the eye, and say, 'Hey, Buddy, could you spare a buck?' Now, I don't waste no time with that nickel and dime stuff. Most hits get me twenty bucks or a ten spot, at least."

"What is the importance of getting in step?"

"I've found that bluntly interruptin' a person gets you nowhere. I don't know. It's like maybe they feel I'm more like them, just not as lucky as they are, ya know. Most people seem to identify with me when I've walked along beside them for a while. They have a tough time tellin' me 'no.'"

"You mentioned that you have been involved in some frightening situations."

"Oh, yeah. Let me give ya an example. I'm thinkin' it was Christmas Eve. I hit on a guy that seemed like a pretty good target. Man! Was I ever wrong! I ended up bein' the target because he must of been watchin' me havin' a super day. That guy pushed me into the alley and threatened to punch my lights out if I didn't give him all my dough! He kept mumblin' that he hated to do it, but that he could tell I was a pro, and his kids weren't gonna have Christmas unless he took my money. He kept sayin', 'She's makin' me do it! She's makin' me do it!' When I asked him, 'Who's makin' you do it, man?' He said, 'It's all my wife's fault! She's driven me to drink, and I can't keep a steady job.' You know, he played the part of the victim real good. I wanted to give him a lecture, but he was too strung out to listen."

"What would you have told him?"

"I was wantin' to say, 'Man, I used to feel sorry for myself, ya know? Then I got to figurin' out who had been makin' all those dumb choices in my life, and it was me. We make our own luck, and no one can make us do anything. We are always responsible for our actions.'"

"That is profoundly stated, Joe. My next question is a difficult one for me to ask. Do some people accuse you of being a freeloader?"

"Yeah, I've really struggled with that one, especially when my mother starts cryin' about how she wished I'd gone into the family business, ya know? I tell her I'm a pattern-buster. I can live off my inheritance from my dad, but I just can't follow my grandpa's or my dad's path. I gotta make my own choices. I gotta be me!"

"You have been called a modern day Robin Hood.

Why is that?"

"Ya know, I guess ya could say I give people a chance to feel good about themselves by givin' to others. I ain't never hurt nobody in all these years, and maybe I've done some good. I've always given to those who really need it, especially to a home in our neighborhood for abused kids. It's called Nobility House — it's a safe environment where kids can regain their self-esteem and remember their noble spirit. I've got a real soft spot for these kids."

"Part of your book is about how you get in step with abused children. Will you tell us how you do that?"

"Well, these kids are scared to death of everybody, and you can't even put your hand on their shoulder, ya know? I get in step with 'em just like I do when I'm pan-handlin'. I just be with 'em awhile — sit like they do, don't say nothin' till they do, even breathe like 'em. Pretty soon they start askin' me my name and warm up to me. Then we talk and get to be friends. They call me Uncle Joe. I take 'em to the movies, stuff like that. They learn to trust me 'cause I'm not a threat to 'em."

"Joe, I honor your courage to be your own person. Thank you for sharing your story with us.

*"Our next guest is well known for her research at Harvard University in the field of communications, specializing in rapport. Author of six books, her latest is entitled **Mirror, Mirror, on the Wall Street**. Please welcome Dr. Johanna Powers."*

"Hello, Maya, Joe. What a thrill to be a guest on your first 'High Performance Adventure!'"

"Thank you, Johanna. I am excited about this opportunity. How would you explain Joe's art of getting in step with people?"

"Very simply, Joe is an expert at creating rapport. And rapport is the doorway to successful verbal communications."

"How do you define rapport?"

"Rapport is exactly what Joe calls it — getting in step with another person. It's having a relationship that is harmonious. Rapport creates trust because we like and trust people who get in step with us."

"How do we know when we are in rapport with another person?"

"Here's an example. Everyone please think of a time when you felt that you were really connecting with someone, either in your personal life or in a business situation. From the moment your eyes met, it was as though you were in sync. You both saw things the same way and came to agreement quickly and easily. You were amazed that the words the other person was speaking sounded just like your words. It seemed as though you had known this individual for a lifetime.

"What happened to create this almost instant understanding was the magic of rapport. After these rare occasions, we seem to experience other relationships with a vague dissatisfaction. We know there is a deeper level of communication available, but we're not quite sure how to recapture the magic."

"How do we 'recapture the magic,' Johanna, and make rapport a matter of choice?"

"We need to become more aware of the communications process, so that we do more than merely connect with someone by accident. Let me give you an example. Remember a time when you were walking along and found money on the sidewalk? Maybe it was just a lucky dime, or a quarter, or even a one dollar bill. How did it make you feel? Great? Like someone was looking after you? Like it was going to be your lucky day?

"When I was young, my family visited my grandfather in Holland. Opa was a silver-haired chessmaster, an artist, who loved to go for walks in the park or at the beach in Scheveningen with us. When we kids found lucky 'dubbeltjes' on the sidewalk or in the sand, we would shriek with delight at our unexpected good fortune. Opa's eyes twinkled, lighting up his whole face. In fact, he enjoyed our excitement so much that one day Dad dropped a coin just so we would find it and get all excited. After that, anytime we found a coin, Opa would wink at Dad knowingly as if to say, 'You're the one behind all the fun.'"

"That is an excellent analogy. You are saying that we can plan rapport?"

"Yes, exactly. Rapport is similar to finding lucky money and may happen quite by accident. But with some understanding and a little practice, we can easily be 'the one behind all the fun.'"

"The communications process is enjoyable, once we use the right software programs for our brain/minds. We are going to be constantly referring to ways to make our brains more user friendly on this program by using software for the brain that we call Brainware. How do you recommend that our audience develop Brainware for rapport, Johanna?"

"Rapport creates magic in a relationship and is an easily acquired skill. Since we often slip into rapport unconsciously, the first step is to become more conscious of what is going on when we are communicating with someone. Although psychologists rarely agree with each other, they do agree that the communications process is much more than just the spoken word. Yet when we think of communications, we primarily think of the words we speak.

"Research has shown that on the average only 7 percent of the communications process is the spoken word. The other 93 percent consists of all the unconscious signals that we are constantly sending and receiving."

"What are some of these signals?"

"They are messages that we unconsciously send,

such as our appearance — clothing, height, weight — body posture, facial expressions, gender, race, voice tone and volume, rate of speech, accent, eye movements, even our way of breathing. All of these signals are important to our understanding of the communications process.

"Although our subconscious receives and stores this 93 percent, we're usually not consciously aware of the messages we've received, other than having a vague feeling about someone. We need to make a conscious choice to enter the special state of understanding that builds trust in relationships — the state of rapport.

"Many years ago when I bought my first personal computer, I was a graduate student and didn't have the time to take lessons to learn to be computer literate. As a result, I limped along, trying to figure out what to do by myself. I barely managed to teach myself enough word processing to get me through my research papers.

"Now that I have a computer network with voice-driven PC's, I've taken classes to be able to take advantage of the technology available, especially as it pertains to the area of artificial intelligence. This new understanding has given me a wide range of capabilities that I didn't have previously. It's as though I was barely in the 7 percent communications category before. Now I'm making a conscious choice to understand some of the remaining 93 percent of the communications process with my state-of-the-art equipment."

"How can we become more conscious of the other 93 percent of our communications?"

Joe: "I'll answer that, Maya. It's easy — just pay attention to the other guy's signals and do the same thing. Realize that when you match someone else, you quickly understand exactly how they feel — you get inside their mind."

Johanna: "That's right, Joe. Rapport involves matching or mirroring our communication partner. The best way to observe natural, unconscious mirroring is to watch couples who are in love. Their natural response is to mirror almost every move made by their partner.

"Once we become aware of the rapport process, people-watching can become a fascinating hobby. Pick any restaurant and begin the observation process. As soon as you spot a couple who are engrossed in each other, wait for one of them to take a drink of water, coffee, whatever. Then begin counting. Usually, within seven seconds their partner will also take a drink, if they are in rapport. One of them will lean forward — so will the other. One places their elbows on the table — the other person follows suit. A good relationship can be compared to a dance because of these intricate communications patterns that flow smoothly and effortlessly."

"Are there ways to recognize when we are in rapport, Johanna?"

"Yes. A good way to observe your own rapport process is to do a mental stop-action when you are with someone you care about. From time to time, remind yourself to notice how you and the other person are naturally matching each other. We all do this. Being in rapport is a natural process, directed by our subconscious mind, until we decide to take conscious control over the communications process."

"Rapport Brainware will help our audience make this unconscious process conscious, opening up an important facet of understanding others. Will you give us some examples of rapport, Johanna?"

"Sure. A single friend reported that she was seated next to an attractive man on a flight from Denver to San Francisco. Several attempts to start a conversation with him got nowhere. This woman did not give up, but waited until the meal was served. She then subtly matched almost every move of her neighbor's eating process, and like magic, he began talking with her. They had an interesting conversation during the balance of the flight!

"Another friend, a sales executive named Millie, was talking to me about one of her prospects. She had never been able to set an appointment with this person because he was always too busy to talk with her. When Millie understood rapport techniques, she realized that she had been approaching him in the wrong manner. Millie normally speaks very fast, so she had to slow her rate of speaking to match this prospect, who is from England. She even spoke with a slight British accent the next time she called him, and she immediately got in rapport. As a result, they had a lunch appointment, and her prospect is now a good client. All this occurred because she made the effort to get in step with him."

"Some people in our audience are wondering, 'Isn't matching too obvious?'"

"Effective matching registers the message in the subconscious mind that this is someone like us. We tend to like and trust people who are similar to us. A word of caution, though — matching should be graceful and subtle. It is not an obvious mimicking of others. Mimicking quickly destroys rapport and trust."

"Thank you, Johanna. And now I ask our audience, will the rapport process work for you?"

Audience Member #1: "I know this stuff works, because I recently finished reading one of Dr. Powers' books. It was just in time, too, because my fiance and I got into a fight over an old boyfriend who dropped by to see me. I didn't even let the guy in my apartment. I simply whispered that he had to leave — fast! Of course, my fiance had already seen him and got really jealous and really quiet. So I matched his quietness. After about five minutes of silence, he said, 'Well, I suppose I could get real mad about this, but I don't see that it would do much good.' In similar situations in the past, when he got quiet, I'd start talking. I'd try to get him to talk to me, and then he'd blow up and leave. This time it felt like I was matching him, and we were in rapport. I was finally able to understand his thinking process and where he was coming from. Now I realize that I need to let him experience his feelings in silence, instead of pushing him to talk when he isn't ready. That was the shortest fight we've ever had!"

"Thank you for sharing your experience. Participation from our audience is a vital part of 'High Performance Adventure.' Your seats are equipped with a mini-console that allows us to conduct a poll on various issues. How many of you can identify a specific area of your life in which you need to get in step with another person? If so, please select the button on your console marked 'Yes.'

"I am able to get an immediate reading of total responses on the central monitor. It shows that 99 percent of you responded 'Yes.' Who will give us feedback?"

Audience Member #2: "I need to create a better working relationship with my boss. I don't understand her, but now I can see that I haven't tried very hard to figure out how she sees our relationship."

Audience Member #3: "One of my employees is going through a lot of problems with his family, and these problems are affecting his productivity on the job. I'm going to get in step with him so I can understand him better and help him get through this tough time."

Audience Member #4: "I'm an account executive with a large advertising firm. I plan to get in step with my customers to do a better job of meeting their needs, instead of just trying to close a sale so I can make a big commission."

Audience Member #5: "I'm a single parent, and I've been coming home from work too tired to deal with my two young daughters. I plan to be a better parent by getting in rapport with them. I want to be a good Mom, but I didn't realize how important rapport and understanding are until now."

Audience Member #6: "I'm the 1 percent who said 'No.' I feel it's up to others to get in step with me. That may sound selfish, but that's the way I feel."

"Please tell us why you feel that way."

Audience Member #6: "I guess it's because I don't want to be manipulative and trick other people with some college psychology stuff. If people like me, they like me. If they don't, that's tough! I don't like playing games with people's minds."

"Do you speak Spanish, Russian, French, or any other foreign language?"

Audience Member #6: "Well, I can speak some Spanish."

"Imagine that you have a guest in your home who speaks no English, only Spanish. What language would you speak with this individual?"

Audience Member #6: "Spanish, of course."

"Rapport, getting in step, simply helps us understand each other by speaking the other person's language. It is not manipulative, assuming your motives are honest."

Audience Member #7: "I was raised on a red-dirt farm in Southwest Oklahoma, where I was taught that if I was going to eat, I had to work. And I want to know, how can someone who is no more than a beggar be calling himself successful?"

Joe: "Sir, do you attend church?"

Audience Member #7: "Yeah."

Joe: "Do you put money in the collection plate each Sunday?"

Audience Member #7: "Yeah, I usually tithe my 10 percent. What business is it of yours, anyway?"

Joe: "Does some of that money go to help the poor?"

Audience Member #7: "Yeah, I guess so, but I still don't understand where you're headed."

Joe: "How does it make you feel, helpin' the less fortunate?"

Audience Member #7: "Well, good, I guess. But you can't be calling yourself 'the less fortunate!'"

Joe: "Would you feel better if I was poor and unsuccessful?"

Audience Member #7: "Well, no. I mean, yeah, uh, I guess so."

Joe: "What you're sayin' is you prefer to reward failure over success."

Audience Member #7: "No, I'm certainly not saying that."

Joe: "Yet, that is what you do."

Audience Member #7: "Well ... I'm still opposed to what you do, but I guess I have to admire your understanding of how to get in step with people. There are some areas of my life where I could use some of these ideas."

"Would you please give us an example?"

Audience Member #7: "I have a college-age son I don't understand at all. I always thought it was his fault we don't get along. But maybe it's up to me to get in step with him."

"Thank you for your openness. When you use rapport with your son, it will make a positive difference in your relationship."

Audience Member #8: "My job is in the customer service department of a large department store. About one out of five of my interactions is with a very hostile customer. How do you get in rapport with a person who's out of control?"

Johanna: "That's an excellent question, and I'm glad you brought it up. The answer is deceptively simple —

the opposite of what we've been taught. Sir, how were you trained to handle an angry customer?"

Audience Member #8: "Calm them down, of course."

Johanna: "When you are angry, do you like to be calmed down?"

Audience Member #8: "Not really."

Johanna: "Rapport means being on the same mental plane."

Audience Member #8: "Are you saying I should get angry and shout back at them?"

Johanna: "No, not at all, but you should match their intensity level. Once you let them know your intense concern, you can lead them to a calmer state of mind. Studies show that angry people calm down more rapidly when rapport techniques are used."

Audience Member #8: "That sounds like fun!"

Johanna: "Yes, plus you don't have to internalize so much anger and frustration. Being out of rapport is not healthy for either party. Enjoy this new tool. Expect a new level of success in handling customer complaints."

"Johanna, do you have another example of rapport?"

"Yes, I have a personal story. I was completing a seminar on communicating through rapport and asked the audience for feedback on what they had gained. I received several different answers, and then one very outspoken man stated loudly, 'I want to enroll in your training program!' He was referring to an advanced communications class I was offering. He came up to me after the meeting and started speaking very intensely about some of the problems he was facing. He was almost shouting. There were quite a few people around, so I attempted to maintain rapport while speaking more softly than he, even though I knew better.

"Then he spoke even louder, saying, 'You don't understand me! You don't know where I'm coming from!'

"Deciding to ignore everyone around us, I began

speaking with loud intensity, repeating what he had said he wanted to gain from the class. 'When you get involved in our program, you'll find that your relationships will improve and you'll be more in charge of your life!'

"'Now you understand what I mean,' he said, and he wrote out his check immediately. I didn't match his frustration — just the intensity and volume of his voice, and it worked like magic. Rapport is a valuable tool. Use it and gain new understanding in your relationships!"

"*Thank you, Johanna and Joe, for being our first guests, and to our audience members, for your participation. Today's message is vital to developing your Owner's Manual. Complete understanding of communications in your personal and professional relationships is impossible without the magic of rapport.*

"*It is important to practice Rapport Brainware by using a process of mental imagery. Please begin this exercise by closing your eyes, taking several deep breaths to release tension from your body. Allow your mind to take you to a place of total calm — an ocean of sparkling aqua blue. Imagine the feeling of sand and gentle waves on your bare feet. Feel the ocean breeze, hear the cry of the seagulls, and smell the salty air. Take another deep breath as you relax, enjoying the beautiful setting for a few moments....*

"*Now imagine a future situation that will require rapport. Choose either a professional or a personal relationship. In your mind, see this situation occurring with rapport and understanding between yourself and the other individual. Feel yourself comfortably matching your communication partner. Hear the words that you both are saying. Enjoy the acceptance, the agreement, the trust.*

"*Repeat the experience by putting yourself fully in the*

scene. See your partner's positive reactions as you purposely establish rapport. You are choosing to create an attitude of acceptance. Enjoy the new understanding you gain by getting in step easily, naturally....

"When you are ready, bring your awareness back to the present time and space, with the knowledge that it is within your power to dramatically enhance your relationships through the use of Rapport Brainware. Repeat this mental imagery a minimum of twice a day, and look forward to obtaining positive results.

"How important is it that you communicate your ideas clearly? How important is it for you to understand what others are communicating? Please join us next week when our topic will be the 'Communications Adventure.' Our guests will include high performers from the world of sports, illustrating how we can understand unconscious communication signals. Look forward to discovering how people process information with their brain/minds from communications specialist, Dr. Paula Edwards. The 'Communications Adventure' will provide you with valuable tools which will help you to become a more powerful communicator.

"This is Maya Cristal, with 'High Performance Adventure.' Use Rapport Brainware, and you will speak the language of understanding."

Announcer: "You may obtain a written transcript of this program and a corresponding Rapport Brainware package by calling the number appearing on your television screen."

Chapter 7

The Dreamtime Connection

Rich rushed onto the dimmed set, "We did it! We did it! Wow! What a start! P. J., you were great. I knew you would be a hit. Johanna, you were brilliant. Maya, what can I say? You're a natural. You're going to be the hottest new star of prime time television to ever emerge from this network — or any network!"

"Thank you for providing the medium to reach many lives, Rich," answered Maya. "But stardom is not what is important. What is important is that people have a genuine commitment to developing their *Owner's Manuals*."

"Would you like to celebrate? Let's catch a late dinner. We can go to the Whole Earth Cafe and ..."

"No, thank you, Rich. It has been a long day. I am going home to my comfortable chair and my cat, Jopie."

"Maya, you are out of this world! How can you be so calm? How can you ignore what's going on here?"

"I am certain you will celebrate enough for both of us. I will call you in two days to let you know what to expect on our next program. And Rich, do not attempt to understand me. Concentrate on understanding your-self."

"Huh? What do you mean by that?"

"Never mind. Good night, Rich."

The traffic moved slowly as Maya's taxi drove south toward her secluded home in the foothills. She leaned back and mentally reviewed the first program. Ignoring the cab driver's blaring radio, Maya closed her eyes and drifted into an alpha state of relaxation. On her mental screen appeared a long, winding, unpaved road leading to a high plateau. She could see fire in the distance. Suddenly the road burst into flames. There was a little girl running toward the flames, while a woman and a man shouted, "Maya, Maya, turn back! It isn't safe!" The little girl stopped, and Maya recognized the child as herself. The little Maya turned around, then slowly disappeared into the smoke.

The images disappeared as Maya heard, "You okay, lady? This is your place, ain't it?"

"Yes, I must have drifted off for a moment. Thank you. Good night."

"Be careful lady. You look awful pale. Watch your step. Don't want no lawsuits."

"Good night."

Δ Δ Δ

Maya held her cat, Jopie, close to her heart, looking into his understanding eyes. She felt disoriented and somewhat lonely. What was the significance of the images she had seen?

I will know soon. I need to get some rest, she thought. Sleep always comes easily for me. I need to use my switching-off procedures again. After a few minutes her brain wave frequency slowed once again to an alpha state.

The winding road reappeared. She could see a woman and a man in the distance, although smoke clouded her view. She walked slowly toward them, cautious but unafraid. The little girl was walking with her — a child Maya and a grown Maya. The child smiled an innocent hello.

"I have been here before? It seems so familiar."

"Yes, you first came here when you were my age. I always knew I would, I mean that you would be on this mission. I am here to lead you back to Mother, Father, and Carlos. This is your first return visit, and they warned me it might be difficult for you to enter your Dreamtime. That taxi episode gave us a scare, though. It would have been most unsafe to get caught between realities again. Forgive me. I am talking too much."

"I am confused. Where are we? Why am I here with myself as a child?"

"You are serious! Carlos told me that this might happen. You are approaching our home in Chichen Itza. The Council has asked Carlos and our parents to advise you during your Dreamtime so that your mission will be flawless. Do you remember?"

"Yes, of course ... now I remember. It was difficult switching to this reality. Earthling encoding is very strong. How much further?"

"When you are ready, stand still and close your eyes."

"I am ready now." Maya closed her eyes, and moments later she heard a familiar voice.

"Welcome back, my sister."

"Carlos, I am glad to see you!" They held each other in a warm embrace. "Where is little Maya?"

"She served you well, but in the future, you should be able to enter your Dreamtime unassisted. We are pleased with your acceptance into the 21st Century. You have accomplished much in a short time. Each trip back will be different. The harmonic frequency is your connection to your destiny. Listen carefully, for your five tones will guide you safely. Without being attuned to this frequency, you could lose your way as you did in the realm of the Dreamstalker."

"Carlos, the Earthlings are a puzzle to me. They are most eager to discover advanced technologies in every field of science except the science of human potential. They are resistant to advances which will increase their personal power. They hold much negativity and live robotic existences — many living with little or no passion for what they are doing. Some have no understanding of their personal power. They do what they are told without questioning. Although they seem quite gifted in the ability to love, they are underdeveloped in the area of understanding."

"Maya, that is why you are there. Your mission will succeed because you are lovingly patient with the Earthlings. The best way to help them is by letting each guest on your program reveal a segment of the *Owner's Manual* so that people will access their own understanding and memory of who they are."

"Thank you, Carlos." The images of her parents appeared before her. "I have missed you, Mother and Father. Did you know the challenge would be this demanding?"

"Yes," replied her mother, "although we prefer to call it rewarding. We love you very much, and we are so proud. All of us in Mayata are aware of your program. It is very entertaining, especially for the older generations. Some remember their writing and final encoding of their *Owner's Manuals*."

Her father cautioned, "When you return to Earthling awareness, you will not be able to remember being with us, but the intuitive feeling will be with you. It will help. Watch for those who realize who you are, for they are special. They will speed your mission toward its ultimate success."

Δ Δ Δ

Maya awoke from a deep sleep. The alarm clock would not stop ringing. Oh ... the phone, she thought, as she reached for it.

"Good morning, Maya. This is Rich. Have you read your morning paper yet?"

"No, Rich, I have not."

"Maya, we're an overnight success! We did it! We did it!"

"Did what?"

"We must have knocked the Neilson's clear out of the sky! You should read the reviews. I knew you could do it. We've got the hottest prime time talk show ever!"

"'High Performance Adventure' has no choice but to be successful."

"You're acting so calm, Maya. Wait until you see your desk — telegrams and fax messages all over the place. People loved P. J. White — want to see more of him. I knew they would! We only got half a dozen or so complaints that he has a dishonest way of asking for handouts, even though the money goes to a good cause."

"That is not at all the point I was emphasizing. Joe is simply a master of rapport."

"I know. I know. No problem. I love the controversy. With ratings like ours, don't worry about what they say — just keep them talking!"

Chapter 8

The Communications Adventure

"*Welcome to 'High Performance Adventure,' the program that helps you maximize your potential through developing an Owner's Manual for your brain. I am your guide, Maya Cristal.*

"Are there times when you wish that you could communicate more effectively with your family members and co-workers? Are there people in your life whom you do not understand?

"Our program this evening will provide you with tools for developing your communication skills and your understanding of how others process their thoughts. We will feature three high performers from the world of sports and communications specialist, Dr. Paula Edwards, from Sydney, Australia, who will introduce tonight's Brainware. Please welcome Dr. Paula Edwards."

"Hello, Maya, and good evening, everyone. It's an honor to be a guest on *the* most talked about program. My friends have been calling to say they can't wait for their next Brainware package from 'High Performance Adventure.' You are a smashing success, Maya!"

"Thank you, Paula. It is exciting to be the host for this program. Our Brainware this evening covers a fascinating area of the communications process which you refer to as the VAK communications system. Please explain this advanced technology."

"VAK is a vital part of the 93 percent of the communications process that, for most of us, is unconscious. As you mentioned last week, only an average of 7% of what we communicate is our spoken words. Once our audience becomes fluent in using the VAK Brainware package, they will be amazed at their increased understanding."

"What does VAK represent?"

"These are the visual, auditory, and kinesthetic sensory systems which our brains constantly use to send and receive information. We use all three of these sensory systems, but we usually have a preferred system, which is called our primary system."

"Will you give us a brief description of each system? Our audience will receive more detail in the complete Communications Brainware package."

"Before I go into the descriptions, I want to say something about eye-accessing cues that are common to each system. Our eyes are neurologically connected to our brains, which means that when we process thoughts, we usually move our eyes in specific ways to help us retrieve information quickly and efficiently. This use of our eyes has been carefully studied and categorized according to the VAK communications system. When we become aware of how people are accessing information with their eyes, we will know a great deal more about them, and thus the 93 percent communications process becomes more conscious."

"Tell us about these eye-accessing cues."

"Most people are patterned in a standard manner. A few are 'wired' differently, and the way to understand a person's eye-accessing patterns is to calibrate their eye movements.

"For visual accessing of remembered information, called visual recall, answer the question, 'What did your room look like when you were ten years old?' If you noticed the direction that your eyes moved, most of you looked up and to the left."

"What eye movements correspond to visualizing an imaginary event?"

"We call that visual construct. For example, 'What would a cat look like with green fur?' Most of you will find that you looked up and to the right.

"To demonstrate auditory recall, answer the question, 'What does your favorite song sound like?' The auditory accessing cues follow the same directions as visual, except the movement of the eyes is horizontal. Most of you moved your eyes to the left. For auditory construct, 'What would a Martian's voice sound like?' The eye-accessing cue is horizontal and to the right. There's another cue for when we talk to ourselves. For example, 'Why didn't I tell her exactly what I was thinking?' The eyes usually travel down and to the left.

"And when we get into our feelings, we are in the kinesthetic system, 'What would you feel like if you were called into your manager's office and reprimanded?' The eye-accessing cue is usually down and to the right.

"Children demonstrate kinesthetic eye movements best. When you scold children, where do their eyes automatically go? Down, of course, because they are experiencing their emotions. Often an irate parent will scold their child and then say, 'Look at me when I'm talking to you.' That doesn't allow the child space to experience her feelings."

"What will awareness of these eye accessing cues mean to our audience?"

"The VAK communications system is a vital part of developing rapport. Once we are aware of a person's primary system, we can quickly get in step with them by choosing to communicate in that system."

"Paula, please describe the different systems in more detail."

"Certainly, Maya. Let's start with people whose primary system is visual. These people are constantly making pictures on their mental screen. You can recognize them because they often try to speak as fast as their rapidly changing images. To others, the primary visual seems to talk too fast.

"When primary visuals, PV's, look up and stop talking, they are viewing the myriad of pictures in their minds. One way to honor their thinking process is not to interrupt them. Our impulse is to speak when our communication partner is silent because we are uncomfortable with the silence and want to fill the void. Don't. It will break rapport.

"PV's usually take more shallow breaths than other sensory systems. They breathe from high in their chests, which makes their tone of voice high and even shrill, especially when they get excited."

"How else can we recognize primary visuals?"

"Listen for the visual words — 'see, look, picture, view, imagine, appear.' PV's love lots of visual aids in presentations. The more visuals they have, the better. They also love color — colorful descriptions, colorful homes and offices, colorful clothes. They like to accumulate things, which makes them the world's most dedicated shoppers. You can also recognize PV's by the neatness of their home and office. Although everything may not always be in its place, they would like it to be because untidiness disturbs them. PV's also have a tendency to suffer from shoulder and neck tension due to their constant straining to see images. This is just a brief summary of PV traits, and these are very general traits. It's important to remember that no two people are exactly alike."

"We will be more effective when we communicate with primary visuals by honoring their world — by using visual words and visual examples."

"Yes. When we match someone's communications system, we are building rapport. The key is to increase our awareness of the 93 percent of the communications process that is usually unconscious."

"Thank you, Paula.

"It is time to introduce a guest who is a colorful example of a primary visual. At age seventy-five, she states that she is in the best physical condition of her life. She is a marathon runner, a clothing designer, and calls herself an environmental activist. Please welcome Lois Campbell."

"Hello, Maya, Dr. Edwards. It's good to **see** you."

*"Thank you, Lois. You certainly are a high performer. Please give us some **insight** into your life."*

"Well, I have several passions in life. One of them is running. Another is the line of **colorful** activewear I design and market. And I have a third passion which I'll describe later."

"How did you develop a passion for running?"

"When I turned forty, I **saw** myself starting a downward spiral. Just little things — bulges here and there — little aches and pains. My mother had left me with the **impression** that I needed to accomplish whatever I wanted by the time I turned forty, because from there on, it was all downhill! Can you **imagine** that? I was living the grim **picture** she had **painted** for me, until one day I woke up! The doctors wanted to perform surgery for a malignant growth, and I said, 'No!' I **saw** my health as my own responsibility. I read everything I could on healing and wellness and started **visualizing** myself as the **picture** of perfect health. I also changed my diet and began my running program."

"Were you able to avoid surgery?"

"Absolutely. The doctors couldn't **see** how it had happened, but I experienced total remission from the cancer."

"You took no drugs or cancer therapy?"

"Well, I thought about taking radiation treatments at first, but I couldn't **see** myself submitting to the treatments or having surgery — although surgery is necessary in some cases because everyone's different. People must do what's right for them. I found a holistic doctor who worked with me to heal the cause of the tumor. I made changes in my lifestyle, and I also **saw** how dysfunctional programs had been running my life for years. I worked to eliminate these negatives from my life. My doctor also recommended a change in diet and advised me to take certain nutritional supplements. She taught me to use mental **imagery** in my healing process. I spent two, sometimes three, fifteen-minute periods a day **visualizing** myself completely healed."

"Please explain this process."

"First, I put myself into a relaxed state by mentally **seeing** myself on a beautiful mountainside. Then I **pictured** the cancer cells in my body being erased by the white blood cells, which I **saw** as giant erasers. Next, I **visualized** myself leaving the doctor's office after being told I was totally free of cancer. I could even **see** the doctors shaking their heads in confusion over my miraculous remission. Well, it took about six months before my **images** became a reality, and I've had no trace of cancer since. That was over thirty years ago."

"Congratulations on taking responsibility for your wellness. Have you continued to run?"

"Oh, yes! I started slowly and kept on building my strength. Then I got this **picture** in my mind of running to the top of a mountain and back. It was like I was already there. I began to train seriously for the race up Pikes Peak. Of course, my time didn't break any records, but I did that race more than once. I still run the trail at least once a month in the summer, but my knees have let me know to slow down a bit."

"What is the length of the trail?"

"It's thirteen miles."

"It must take planning, preparation, and endurance to do what you have done."

"Yes, it does. It really helps to know that before I even start to run, in my mind, I **see** that I've already arrived. I can **picture** myself at the top, and that **image** keeps me running."

"Tell us about your design business."

"When I first started running, I couldn't find running apparel that **looked** right to me. So I bought some new wonder fabrics with built-in stretch and made my own activewear. I got bored with the solid-colored fabrics and started designing some **colorful** prints, drawing from my love of nature. You will **see** the pieces in activewear shops and boutiques all over the country."

"Is that one of your designs you are wearing?"

"Yes. Some of my designs honor endangered species. You **see**, I consider myself an environmental activist, because whatever I can do to increase the **visibility** of this issue and raise the awareness of others, I want to do it. The golden eagle on this quilted jacket is hand-painted. The running tights and T-shirt pick up the **green**, **brown**, and **gold colors** of the Earth that I **imagine** the eagle must **see** from her **perspective**. Along with that, I've added the **blue** of the sky. When I run in this, I **see** the world from the eagle's point of **view**. It's almost like I'm flying over the ground."

Paula: "You must feel very proud of your accomplishments, Lois."

Lois: "Well, Dr. Edwards, I can **see** that my life is just beginning. Next month I'm starting a lecture tour. After that ..."

Paula: "It's interesting that Lois responded to my 'feel' question with a visual word."

Lois: "I did? I guess you're right. Feelings run deep with me, but it's easier for me to describe how things **appear** to me."

Paula: "When we agree on a subject, there is no problem in using different communications systems. But let me ask you, Lois. You must have felt a lot of anger and fear when the doctors diagnosed you as having cancer."

Lois: "No, not really. I just refused to **see** things their way."

Paula: "But what were you feeling?"

Lois: "**Look**, Dr. Edwards, I'm totally comfortable with my feelings. I just **looked** at it as a challenge, a time in my life to make choices. I'm very happy with who I am."

Paula: "I apologize, Lois. I can **see** you have been offended by my probing questions. I can also **see** that you are proud of your accomplishments and rightfully so. I was hoping our audience would get the **picture** of the miscommunications that can occur when we don't match a person's primary communications system."

Lois: "I didn't think you **saw** where I was coming from just a moment ago."

Paula: "Exactly the point I'm making. When we use a different system from that of our communication partner, it can cause a conflict — because we're speaking different languages."

Audience Member #1: "My son is an oncologist, and he's told me of numerous cases of people who thought their cancer was cured, but it really wasn't. He says that people are just fooling themselves with all this visualization and self-healing nonsense. I think people who don't put themselves totally under a doctor's care are crazy!"

Lois: "My doctor has taught me that there's a big difference between healing a disease and curing it. Healing deals with the cause of our illness, which means we must correct the imbalance in our lives that made us sick. Curing just deals with the symptoms, such as having surgery to cut out a tumor. It may come back if we don't deal with the cause.

"My doctor is willing to share my x-rays with others. She can't explain it, but she has to admit I'm clean."

Audience Member #2: "I also have a question for Lois Campbell. Your statement about being an environmentalist sounds pretty radical to me, but I bet you live by a double standard. You probably enjoy a nice steak, and don't mind killing animals for food, like the rest of those eco-hypocrites!"

Lois: "As a matter of fact, I'm a vegetarian. I eat no red meat, chicken, or fish. However, I do not campaign against the humane killing of animals, if it's part of a food chain. I do have a problem with the inhumane testing of chemicals and cosmetics on laboratory animals and the cruel trapping of animals by the fur industry."

Audience Member #2: "Just as I thought — another radical."

Lois: "It's not my intent to be a threat to anyone. I simply honor all forms of life. You have absolutely nothing to fear from an environmental activist! Societies that honor the Earth and her animal inhabitants have been around for many thousands of years. Societies that believe they have total dominion over the Earth and can freely use up her resources have been around for only two hundred years. The results are obvious. Future generations will **view** us 'radicals' as saviors of their planet."

*"Thank you, Lois, for giving us a **glimpse** into your **colorful** lifestyle.*

"Paula, will you explain our next communications category?"

"Certainly. Let's talk about the primary kinesthetic group. These PK's prefer to process their thoughts kinesthetically — that is, through their feelings and also through touch, taste, and smell. They are easy to recognize because they speak more slowly and at a lower pitch than visuals. Feelings take longer to process than pictures, so when a PK breaks eye contact to look down and to their right, do not interrupt their thought processing. They will look at you when they are ready to continue the conversation. Because of their slower speech, PK's are sometimes thought of by PV's as being mentally slow, but that's not the case. They are simply processing information differently from visuals.

"PK's can also be identified by their frequent use of feeling words such as 'feel, touch, warm, soft, grasp, hold, sense, and connect.' These individuals are the huggers of the world. They love to touch and be touched."

"There must be frequent communication breakdowns between visual and kinesthetic partners."

"Absolutely. Because they process information so very differently, a PV and a PK who are married, or who work together, need to understand each other's sensory systems. Let me give you an example. One of my friends, a raving visual, has a very kinesthetic husband. When she comes home from a long day at work, she wants to show Jim that she loves him by taking him out to dinner. It also would mean a great deal to her if Jim sent her flowers more often and paid attention to the little things that show her that he loves her. Now Jim is perfectly satisfied to spend the evenings, sitting on the couch, holding Marian and feeling that she loves him.

"Their differences have created a great deal of conflict and miscommunications in the past. Now that they are both aware of their preferred sensory systems, Jim is conscious of showing Marian how much he loves her, and Marian makes every effort to communicate her love for Jim through touch. In fact, because she talks so fast, she slows down when she's making an important point with Jim, and may touch his hand or put her arm around him. In the past, she would rattle off a request and become frustrated when it didn't even register with him. Their relationship has grown much stronger because they are using their VAK understanding."

"Thank you, Paula.

"Our next guest is Kenny Johnson, the offensive left tackle for the Denver Broncos and winner of last year's NFL Sportsmanship Award. Welcome to our program, Kenny."

"Hi, Maya. I **feel** like it's a real, uh, honor to be on your show."

"Thank you, Kenny. In a recent interview with **Sports Today,** *you stated that the game of football was the closest thing to heaven for you. Please explain why you* **feel** *that way."*

"Well, ever since I was a little kid, I've **felt** strongly about football, you know. I, uh, had this older brother who played ball in high school and got a scholarship to Nebraska, but well ... he never got to play."

"What happened?"

"Well, uh, he was killed in a car wreck right before he was supposed to leave for college. He, you know, he was my idol."

"Did you decide to play football because of your **feelings** *for him?"*

"Yeah. I **felt** like I had to be the best, uh, for Johnny.

Often, in the **heat** of the game, when everything is **flowin'** smoothly, I can, you know, **feel** like he's right there with me."

"What do you like best about the game?"

"Well, I guess it would have to be the **feeling** of playing my best and winning."

*"Over the years, there has been much talk about athletes using drugs such as **pain** killers, muscle relaxers, and antibiotics to allow them to play with injuries. I understand you have a unique way of handling **pain**."*

"Well, uh, I've always refused to take any drugs. I've **felt** it just wasn't worth the risk to my mind and body, you know? My body just seems to heal faster when I, uh, don't mask the **pain** with drugs. I **feel** I can play through any injury by remembering what it **felt** like before I, uh, got hurt. I just hold on to the good **feeling**."

*"You are known **affectionately** among your team members as 'Big Brother.' Why?"*

"Well, I guess it's 'cause I **care** a lot about the rookies and try to keep 'em from messin' up, you know, with drugs, and all that stuff. It takes a while for kids to get a **grasp** on what the real world's all about. And, uh, you know, I try to be there for them."

"Kenny, what has been the key to your success?"

"Oh, I guess I've always **felt** that there was no challenge too great for me to accept. You always hear guys mention peakin' out, but I never **felt** that way. I **feel** that my commitment to do my best, uh, has gotten me a long way. Also, I **feel** like I've, uh, always been in the right place at the right time. You know, I've always, **grabbed** every opportunity that came along and gone for it."

*"What do you **feel** would be good advice for our audience that will help them be more effective as high performers?"*

"Get **in touch** with your **feelings** so that you can be the best ... and then act on your **feelings**. It doesn't do any good to get all **pumped up** and then do nothin' with all that **excitement**. The high performers in this world, I don't **care** what field they're in — sports, business, whatever — the winners are the ones that, uh, you know, go out and make things happen!"

"Thank you, Kenny, and best wishes for a successful season."

Audience Member #3: "Maya, I feel betrayed by your apparent approval of brutal contact sports."

"Please tell us why you feel this way."

Audience Member #3: "My son went out for football, like all of his friends. He loved it — couldn't talk about anything else every day when he came home from practice. Then, one day, he didn't come home ..."

"What happened?"

Audience Member #3: "He was killed during a routine practice session. He had a concussion and died of internal hemorrhaging."

"I feel your pain and bitterness."

Audience Member #3: "You're damn right, I'm bitter! It was such a useless waste, a crime against his youth and our family. Someone should have warned us about the risks involved, and now it's too late for him. But it's not too late to warn other unsuspecting parents that it could happen to their child, too."

"Awareness of the risks involved seems reasonable, as does freedom of choice. What about the benefits of athletic programs?"

Audience Member #3: "It doesn't matter what good they do. It doesn't balance out the maiming, and it doesn't bring my son back."

Kenny: "You know, my brother was killed by ... a drunk driver. But I **felt** ... that I had to let go of my anger or it would have destroyed me. Also, there's, you know, far more danger in riding in a car than there is in, uh playing football. I **feel,** uh, real sorry about what happened to your son. The odds against such a thing are, you know, really high."

Audience Member #3: "Oh, how can you defend your barbaric sport! All you're doing is defending violence. Odds don't count when it's my son. I hate your kind!"

"What is your hate going to accomplish?"

Audience Member #3: "I can't forgive them."

"What is your hate going to accomplish?"

Audience Member #3: "Maybe I can help to save someone else's son."

"Is hate going to do that?"

Audience Member #3: "Well, maybe not.... I'm not really sure ..."

"I applaud your courage to voice your beliefs. Your life will take on new meaning when you release the hate that you feel. As long as you hold the hatred and bitterness in your heart, you will not heal your emotional wounds. You have mentioned risks. Risk love. Risk understanding. It is your choice.

"Paula, please describe our next communications category."

"Auditories, PA's, are our third category. These individuals prefer to process information by sound. You may recognize them by their love of music and by their love of conversation. They can be heard humming tunes or talking to themselves, although they would rather be engaged in conversation with others. They love words — big, long words — and like to make plays on words. Because of their attention to the sound of their voices, they often are the radio announcers and vocalists of the world. You will recognize PA's by their frequent use of words and expressions such as 'jazzed, loud, harmony, rings true;' 'sounds good to me;' 'I hear what you're saying;' 'that clicks for me.' Watch closely for PA's eye signals, which are eyes horizontal to the left and right.

"One of my good friends is a manager for a large high-tech company. Some people think she has deplorable eye contact because her eyes dart from side to side as she processes information. I always give her the opportunity to hear how an idea sounds by being silent when she breaks eye contact."

"Thank you, Paula.

"Our final guest is the world-renowned tennis champion, winner at Wimbledon for the last three years. Please welcome Elise Hampden."

"Hello, Maya. I've been **hearing** so much about your show, even before I got the invitation to **speak** on your program tonight."

*"Thank you, Elise. Please **tell** us the secret that has kept you a high performer for so many seasons."*

"Well, I've always **heard** that hard work and determination are the keys to success. I've never let anything stop me from believing in myself — in my ability to consistently **ring** the cash register."

"Do you use mental rehearsal to prepare for a match?"

"Yes. What really helps the most is when I **hear** my name being announced as the champion over and over in my mind. While I'm practicing in my mind, I **hear** the announcer, **listen** to the cheering of the crowd, and **hear** the **sound** of my racquet slamming the ball, that sort of thing. It seems like something **clicks**, and my confidence is exactly where I need it to be — supporting me in doing my absolute best."

"You have a phenomenal service return rate. To what do you attribute this ability?"

"Some people have accused me of having bionic **ears**. I can usually **tell** what kind of spin a serve is going to have because of the way the ball **sounds** when the racket hits it."

*"How did you learn to be this accurate in your **hearing**?"*

"It just came naturally, I guess. That's the way I've always played.

"Oh, I've got to tell you — I **heard** a great expression the other day that really **sounded** good to me. It said, 'Life's a piano. The **tune** you **hear** depends on how you play it.'"

*"You are playing a wonderful **song**, Elise. Best wishes for a successful tour.*

"Paula, do you have some additional comments?"

"Yes, Maya. I want to stress that no one falls into just one communications category. We are all a combination of the three VAK sensory systems. In fact, there is a fourth category, which is visual-kinesthetic. These VK's process information by first seeing it, then checking the information with their feelings. Look for the combination of visual and kinesthetic eye cues and listen for the signal words. One of my clients is highly visual, yet also very much in touch with his emotions. He relates easily to both PV's and PK's. The other day he said, 'I'm so pleased with how things are **looking** and **feeling**.'

"The goal of understanding the VAK communications system is to have a balance of the three systems and be able to communicate easily with others, using the words from their preferred system. Again, it is a vital part of rapport to match the sensory language our communication partner is using, which means we use 'see' words with primary visuals, 'sound' words with primary auditories, and 'feeling' words with primary kinesthetics. Use this advanced form of understanding, and you will greatly increase the quality of your personal and professional relationships."

Audience Member #4: "Can you give us another practical use for VAK?"

Paula: "Yes. Knowing how to use VAK understanding can help us resolve conflicts. Let me explain by having everyone think of an argument that you had recently with your spouse, a child, or a co-worker. In your mind, put yourself back in the situation, replaying what happened from your perspective. Visualize what was happening vividly, listen carefully to what you and the other person said, and experience the emotions from your perspective. When you're seeing the event from your eyes, we call this being fully associated with what happened.

"Now go back to the same conflict, putting yourself in the other person's place and reliving what happened. This second viewing of the scene should have given you some new insight into the situation.

"Now take it one step further, this time, replaying what happened as you observe yourself and the other person interacting. We call this disassociating from the event. Visualize the scene, hear what you both said, and watch both of you experiencing your emotions. You have become an observer to the event. This tool of disassociation can be used any time we want to gain a different perspective, or when we want to diminish the power of an event to affect us.

"We can also change the impact of an event by making our memory of it more or less vivid, increasing or decreasing the volume of what was said, and increasing or decreasing the intensity of the emotions. For example, we all know people who think their lives are miserable. Quite frequently, it's because of the way they are viewing the events in their lives. They replay all their unpleasant movies, fully associated, reliving every depressing moment, over and over, in living color. On the other hand, people who are happy and optimistic are replaying their positive movies, rather than the negative ones.

"Let's experience what I'm describing. Think of an unpleasant situation. Replay the scene, from your point of view, fully associated. Make the pictures you are visualizing even more vivid, by turning up the brightness. It might be helpful to imagine that you're in the control room for the movies of your mind, and in front of you is an instrument panel from which you can control these movies.

"Now increase the size of the pictures, and turn up the volume. How does that feel? Probably not too good. Next take yourself out of the picture by disassociating from it.... Now turn the movie into a still shot, and make the picture normal size. Continue decreasing the size until it's the size of a postage stamp. Next, turn down the brightness of the colors until your picture is black and white. Decrease the volume until you finally turn it off. Then take the tiny picture and move it so far behind you that it is no longer visible.... When you're ready, open your eyes."

"Who would like to share your experience of this process?"

Audience Member #4: "That was fun! When I disassociated from my movie, I automatically lost all the volume. This is going to help when bad experiences come back to haunt me!"

Audience Member #5: "I liked it too, but I never could move it behind me. Instead I shrunk my postage-stamp picture into a tiny black dot, and I just erased it. I feel a lot better about the situation now."

Audience Member #6: "When I was replaying my conflict situation, I didn't get any new information. I just felt, more than ever, that I was right!"

Paula: "That's fine. It's okay to be right, but at least give yourself a chance to discover any information that might help you resolve the conflict."

Audience Member #7: "That's what happened to me.

I was able to see a solution that I hadn't considered before. This tool will help me to facilitate closure on some negative experiences with some peers."

Audience Member #8: "I've been in therapy for the last five years to learn to get in touch with my emotions. I don't like this exercise because it seems like a defense mechanism to me."

Paula: "I'm glad you mentioned that. Defense mechanism implies denial of a situation. Using this technique, you have the option to choose how you want to experience your past. There is a big difference between choice and denial."

Audience Member #9: "I don't get all this visualizing stuff. I couldn't come up with any pictures at all."

Paula: "Not everyone has a highly developed visual channel, but you can learn to develop this ability. Simply pretend that you are seeing pictures, and continue to practice. Before long, you will begin to visualize. Also, for some people, it's easier to visualize with your eyes open, looking at the ceiling. You can keep them open to get your images started, and then close them as you gradually develop your visualization skills.

"Let's take this exercise to its completion by substituting a positive experience for the unpleasant one. Think of a positive experience that you would like to relive. Begin to replay your movie, noticing if you're fully associated. Some people miss most of the fun in life by observing their pleasant movies from a distance, rather than being fully associated. Turn up the brightness control so that the scenes are in brilliant color. Increase the size, bringing the movie right in front of your face. Next, turn up the volume to a comfortable level, and intensify the feelings, so that you fully experience this event. Enjoy this for a few moments.... When you're ready, open your eyes."

"Who would like to give us your feedback?'

Audience Member #10: "Wow! That was great. I might never want to go to work, just run my best movies over and over!"

Paula: "Please stay in touch with reality, but make it your best reality. It's all a matter of choice. Do we choose to replay all our unpleasant experiences over and over and make ourselves depressed? Or do we choose to diminish their impact by using this tool, and then substitute a pleasant experience? One word of caution, the goal is to be fully present in each moment, so we don't want to spend our lives running old movies. Yet, when thoughts come into our minds, we can choose to control them and to control our experience."

Audience Member #11: "This visualization garbage is too much for me! I just think we are what we are, and we should leave it at that."

"Tell me, do you use a computer?"

Audience Member #11: "Of course! Everyone does."

"When your software is updated by the manufacturer, what do you do with the updated programs?"

Audience Member #11: "I install them on my computer. What are you getting at?"

"The Brainware we are offering you is similar to your updated software. The difference is that this program is for your brain/mind. Can you imagine not installing your updated Brainware? This program offers you choices. The old ways are still available to you, and now you have the new understanding available, if you choose to take advantage of it."

Audience Member #12: "Maya, I'm caught between two belief systems. I believe that mental rehearsal works in athletics, and several of my friends have achieved their goals by using mental rehearsal. My problem is that I guess you could say I'm a 'recovering Catholic.' The priest taught us, 'An idle mind is the Devil's workshop.' He said that when we meditate without a specific purpose, then evil spirits can enter our body. In other words, if we meditate to still our minds, or to simply relax, we could be opening our soul to the Devil. Does this make sense to you?"

"Any belief becomes reality the moment it is accepted. This specific belief is a fallacy because the mind must be stilled in order to sleep. Therefore, at least once a day, evil spirits would have free access to your soul. A more functional belief would be to accept evil spirits as powerless unless you give them power over you. Negative or dysfunctional thoughts or spirits exist, as do positive, functional thoughts. It is up to you to choose the thoughts that remain in your mind. It is not magic or voodoo. It is a matter of active choice.

"Thank you, Paula, Lois, Kenny, and Elise, and to each of you in our audience for joining us.

"It is important to take a few moments to practice your Communications Brainware. Please close your eyes, taking a few deep breaths to relax your mind and body. Spend a few moments in your special place — at the ocean, by a stream, in the mountains — that place where you experience total peace of mind....

"Think of a person with whom you want to improve communications. Place yourself in a situation with that person, using your VAK understanding to develop strong rapport. Notice the person's eye-accessing cues, and listen for the words that indicate which system they are using. Now experience what it is like to match them, using the same eye cues and the words that are important to their system. See, hear, and feel yourself having greater understanding of your communication partner than you have had before. Notice that their response is positive and accepting. Experience the pleasure of reaching a new level of trust.

"When you are ready, return your awareness to this space and time, and open your eyes. Repeat your mental

rehearsal at least twice a day, knowing that you have created a blueprint for your success.

"Each brain/mind has a unique method of inputting and retrieving information. VAK Brainware is a communications tool that will increase your understanding of yourself and others. Practice your VAK skills until they become natural.

"Please join us next week for 'High Performance Adventure,' when our topic will be the 'Trust Adventure.' What would it mean to have more trusting personal and professional relationships? How much more effective will you be when you access your Trust Brainware? Our program next week will provide vital information for making your brain user friendly because trust facilitates action. Our guests will be Rama Patel, a successful businessman of the Hindu faith, John McRae and Tom Henson, the United States gold medal champion tandem cycling team, and Laurel Golden and Wayne Mosley-Golden, partnership counselors to business and industry. This is Maya Cristal. Thank you for joining us.

"Remember to add a new dimension of understanding to your communications — speak the language of VAK."

Announcer: "You may obtain a written transcript of this program and a corresponding Communications Brainware package by calling the number appearing on your television screen."

Chapter 9

The Harmonic Frequency

Maya, leaned back in her chair, Jopie purring happily in her lap. The second program had received excellent ratings, and "High Performance Adventure" was on its way. This is just the beginning, she thought. There is much to be done. People must realize that they have at their disposal all that they need to create fulfilling lives for themselves. The *Owner's Manual* is easy to develop. How can people function effectively without it?

Maya closed her eyes and reveled in the perfection of the moment, drifting into an alpha state of consciousness. Moments later, she was aware of the rumble of distant thunder. It is going to rain, yet I am hearing more than just thunder. As a bolt of lightening flashed across the sky, she listened intently. Someone is calling me. Who is whispering my name? I must go.

Feeling no fear, she slipped out into the stormy night. There is something I must do, someone to see, but who? And where? I must follow my heart. I will know soon. She began walking, then running toward the nearby hills. The lightning intensified in a frenzied dance around her — then the rain began.

"Maya, where are you?" She heard a voice close by, then saw a man running toward her.

"Maya, what are you doing out in this storm? Look at you. You're soaked!" Rich exclaimed.

"Oh, Rich, why are you here?"

"Something told me to drive over to make sure you were all right, and then when I saw someone running up the hill, I thought it might be you. Quickly, let's get you home."

"Rich, I must be alone."

"Alone in this place? You're not ready for this!"

"Not ready for what?"

"Please don't question me. I want to see you safely home," Rich insisted.

A brilliant flash of lightning illuminated his face, and in that instant Maya saw a different Rich from the fast-talking television producer. His luminous eyes reflected an understanding that brought the words, "You will not be alone," into her awareness. Intuitively, she knew that she could place total trust in him.

"Very well, Rich. Thank you for your concern."

As Rich dropped her off at her home, she asked, "Would you like to go running with me next week?"

"Sure. Let's run these hills in the daytime!"

A short time later, seated once again in her comfortable chair, she heard, "Maya, Maya, where are you?"

"Who are you? Where are you?" she questioned aloud.

In the midst of the storm she could hear a distinct sound. What was it? Was it music? Then she heard the tones more clearly — five notes sounding over and over, drawing her into their pure harmonic frequency. "I am here. I am waiting," she said. "Who are you?"

"Do you not remember, Maya?"

"Remember what?" She struggled to recapture the pure harmonic tones.

"The harmonic frequency is your connection to your destiny." Who had told her that, and what did it mean?

There it was again. "Maya, remember to be attuned to your tones. You must travel on your harmonic frequency." Slowly, as she stopped struggling to remember, she sensed herself slipping away on the fluid tones, through space and time. Holding persistently to the sounds of harmony, she entered the presence of pure love and understanding. Surrounded by brilliant white light, she again heard her name.

"Maya, you are reaching out to me, as I am to you."

Gradually, a familiar and much-loved image appeared before her. "Oh, it ... it is you, Carlos, my beloved brother!"

"Yes, my sister. I am always ready to receive your transmissions and welcome your presence. This first unassisted connection was your most difficult and dangerous. It is critical that you focus your awareness on your harmonic frequency when you travel in these dimensions. Otherwise, all may be lost. It will be easier for you to reach us as you gradually remember your Galactic powers. Do you bring news?"

"All is going well, Carlos. Already, people are making changes in their lives because of their acceptance that they do have an *Owner's Manual* available to them. I have received many communications from Earthlings who are improving their understanding of themselves and others because they are utilizing their Brainware."

"Yes, Maya. Rapid transformation and change are occurring. It is a time of empowerment for the Earthlings. Their very survival, and that of their Living Spaceship Earth is at stake. It is of great urgency that they understand and act on our message, that in spite of all their so-called advancements, the technology that they value so highly has taken them to the edge of self-destruction. Now they must choose the path beyond technology — the path of the heart. This path will be easier as they develop more trust, a trust and respect that honors the integrity of each individual. They need to understand that they must first trust themselves, and then they will be able to trust others."

"I understand fully, Carlos. Have you completed our mission in Chichen Itza?"

"Yes, hundreds of Earth years have passed since we returned to our Galactic homeland. We are now developing an inter-Galactic communications network for direct transfer of information from Mayata to the Earth plane, as well as to other intelligent life forms occupying planets in this galaxy."

"I look forward to my involvement in this mission after the completion of Mission *Owner's Manual*. Goodbye, Carlos. Goodbye, Carlos. Carlos ... Carlos ... Carlos."

Δ Δ Δ

Maya opened her eyes, murmuring, "Carlos ... Carlos." She did not question the feeling of unconditional love that she experienced as she again consciously repeated, "Carlos ... Carlos."

Chapter 10

The Trust Adventure

"**G**ood evening. This is Maya Cristal welcoming you to 'High Performance Adventure.' Our subject is the 'Trust Adventure,' and our first guest is a high performer in the world of business. Even more important, he represents a way of life that is based on trust — of ourselves and others. Please welcome Rama Patel."

"Namaste, Maya."

"Namaste, Rama. Will you explain to the audience the meaning of our greeting?"

"Quite simply, it is the Hindu greeting, 'I salute the God in you.'"

"When is this greeting appropriate?"

"Any time. All the time. You hear it from those who have many years and from little children. It represents a constant reminder of the divine in each of us."

"Rama, I recently attended a Hindu New Year's celebration. I enjoyed the evening, especially the children's dances and their beautiful ceremonial clothing. I also noticed the attitude of the adults toward the behavior of the young children. They were not sternly disciplined in *the same manner as many American children are."*

"Yes. Each child is treated with respect — as an advanced soul who chooses to be in a child's body. Your Indians, the Native Americans, have a saying, 'Anyone who beats a helpless child is a coward.' We have that same philosophy. My American friends tell me that if you spare the rod, you will spoil the child. Our belief is that if you spank a child once, the child is fearful. The second time, he is again fearful. But the third time, and from then on, he knows what to expect and will go ahead and repeat the offensive behavior. He is thinking, 'I will get spanked, but that's not so bad.' Children and adults fear the unknown much more than the known."

"How many children do you have, Rama?"

"Two little boys, ages five and seven."

"How do you teach them to behave in a manner which is not offensive?"

"Communication is everything — honest, open communication. We must always be truthful. Without truth, it is very difficult to communicate. When we are truthful and reasonable with our children, they will trust us. Inflicting pain on a child only serves to destroy trust.

"I hear parents order their children, 'Do this! Don't do that! I am your father, so you will do as I say.' Instead, I say to my sons, 'I would be very happy if you would do this.' And they do it. It is just that simple because they trust me and want me to be happy."

"That explains why the young children at the celebration were treated with loving tolerance."

"Yes. Tolerance is very important. Any time we point a finger at anyone, we are pointing three fingers at ourselves. So our judgment, blame, intolerance, hatred — all of these harm us much more than the other person."

Audience Member #1: "Rama, I know someone who has just gone to India on a pilgrimage. What is your opinion of such pilgrimages?"

Rama: "I will give my answer in the form of a story. Lord Shiva had a magnificent mango, a very prized and rare variety. Both of his sons wanted to have it. Lord Shiva told them, 'Whoever can go around the world first will receive this prize.' One son started immediately on the long journey. The other son reasoned, 'I know that Lord Shiva is God, who created the world.' So this son walked round his father, and Lord Shiva gave him the mango. What this means is that we don't need to go around the world to find truth. It is right here, within us."

Audience Member #1: "But Rama, I'm very interested in finding out more about your way of life. Can you recommend a good book on Hinduism?"

Rama: "No, no, no, please understand. It is valuable to study a variety of philosophies to give us knowledge and direction, but the real answers are within you. You, yourself are the best book.

"Everything in life is a learning experience. We draw the people and the events in our lives to us because we need to learn something from them."

"Are you saying that even the problems, the difficulties are there because we draw them to us?"

"Yes. My mother, whom I loved very much, died of cancer a few years ago. She did not smoke or drink and ate a strict vegetarian diet, but she constantly put herself under much stress. She worried about me because I was thirty-two before I married. She worried about my sisters — especially the one who became a doctor. Her whole life she worried, and it eventually caused her cancer.

"We believe that all diseases are caused by what we think and how we react to life. Both good and evil are self-imposed."

"Rama, what can the Western world learn from the East?"

"The most important thing is trust. When we trust ourselves, then we are able to be accepting and loving toward others. If we love others and give to them, expecting them to give to us in return, then that is not love — that is commerce. If we treat others with anything other than love, we will create unhappiness for ourselves. We have an important saying, 'Love plus understanding equals happiness. Hatred plus intolerance equals disaster.'"

Audience member #2: "Are you saying we should love everyone — even our enemies?"

Rama: "Yes. We do not make enemies out of enemies. We only make enemies out of friends. Remember, we must love without expectation. Otherwise we don't have love — we have a business arrangement."

Audience Member #3: "How can you say we don't need to read a book to find truth? The only truth is in the Bible!"

Rama: "I have heard it said that the truth shall set you free. Whenever any book claims to have all the answers, then those who believe totally in that theory are not free, but slaves to their book. We have a saying, 'To know the known is to keep the unknown hidden.' The people of the Western world need to open their minds to allow for the unknown, to not limit themselves to narrow definitions. For example, you have a mountain. There is more than one way to get to the top of that mountain — many ways. So it is with truth. There are many paths to truth. Whenever we judge another, we are only hurting ourselves. Judgment means lack of understanding."

Audience Member #3: "I still believe the Bible, 100 percent, no exceptions. It was written by men who were divinely inspired by God."

Rama: "That must be comforting. One question: Which of the over two hundred translations of the Bible do you believe 100 percent?"

Audience Member #3: "That's doubletalk! If it's in the Bible, I believe it!"

Rama: "I perceive that people in the Western world are entirely too serious about themselves and their religion. One day, I saw a humorous saying on a sign which a blind man was carrying. It said, 'Don't worry. If you are well, you don't need to worry. If you get sick, you may die, and if you go to heaven, you won't need to worry. If you go to hell, all your friends will be there. So, don't worry.'"

Audience Member #4: "What is all this nonsense about trust? The last time I trusted someone, it was one of my employees, and they ripped me off for fifty thousand dollars!"

Rama: "Trust does not mean sacrificing rational thinking. We should maintain our awareness at all times."

Audience Member #5: "I've also had a problem with trust. I've been afraid to trust anyone in a relationship, because five years ago I fell in love with my ideal man. We were talking about marriage, when I found out that he was already married and had two kids! He had lied to me about everything, and he destroyed my faith in people."

"Who destroyed your faith?"

Audience Member #5: "He did!"

"What part did you play in the relationship?"

Audience Member #5: "I was taken advantage of."

"Did you make a choice to enter the relationship?"

Audience Member #5: "Well ... yes, I suppose I did."

"Then it was your choice to become involved with this person. No one does anything to us without our permission.

"Every person — every event that we draw to us is our mirror. I suggest that you ask yourself how that

individual was your mirror. When you understand the lesson, then you will be able to release the experience and choose to trust again."

Audience Member #6: "I respect the wisdom of your way of life, Rama, except for one thing. Where does equality for women come into a caste system such as yours?"

Rama: "Ah, that is a good question. There is no equality because Hindu men consider women to be superior to them, and we place the women in our lives on a pedestal."

Audience Member #6: "You've got to be kidding. Your pedestal is nothing short of bondage! What kind of a life is it to be barefoot, veiled, and pregnant?"

Rama: "There is opportunity for women to have a career. For example, my sister is a physician and makes more money than her husband."

Audience Member #7: "I would like to comment on this issue. My homeland is India. Seven years ago I came to this country to attend M.I.T. I now have my doctorate in physics and am employed as a research scientist. My sisters in my country are beginning to awaken to the fact that there is more for them than being on a pedestal. I will return to India in two years to open my own company and give opportunities to women to enter the business world."

Audience Member #6: "Thank you. I just wanted to make sure people are aware that women in countries such as India need their *Owner's Manuals,* also."

"Thank you for your participation. Rama, what message would you like to leave with our audience?"

Rama: "There is a story of Mahatma Gandhi. One day, as the train on which he was a passenger stopped in a village, he was mobbed by the crowd, all asking for a message to take home to their people. He simply said, 'I am my message.' Much more important than what we say is who we are and what actions we take. That is the true message that either inspires trust or destroys it.

"Maya, you asked what the Western world could learn from the East. Another question might be, 'What can the Eastern world learn from the West?' My answer is simple: Action! Action! Action! Eastern philosophy often does not transfer from the heart to the feet. The perfect balance is truth in action.

"Many Americans are embracing Eastern philosophy, and I need to caution that while meditating for many hours may bring heightened awareness, it does not bring about action. It is very important that we put our beliefs into action!"

"Thank you for joining us, Rama, and for sharing your way of life. You are your message.

"Our next guests are high performers, John McRae and Tom Henson, the United States gold medal champion tandem-cycling team. Please welcome Tom and John."

Tom: "It's great to be here, Maya. I really enjoy your show."

"Thank you, Tom. I have been looking forward to meeting both of you. Trust must be vital for you."

"Yes, trust allows me to survive. If I didn't trust people, I'd be dead. I've been blind since birth, but that's never stopped me from leading an active life."

"How did you meet each other?"

John: "My bike had just been stolen, and Tom, who had a bike, was looking for a cycling mate, so it seemed natural to team up."

"Tom, what influenced your becoming a cyclist?"

Tom: "My uncle Michael used to call me a dreamer, and he taught me to dream big. He always told me that we can make wonderful things happen when we put our dreams into action. He taught me to believe in my potential. He used to say, 'Just because you have this handicap doesn't mean you can't achieve greatness. You are blessed with ears that hear better than most, and you can sense things that most people don't sense.' Then a few years ago, he bought me a tandem bicycle. I will always remember my first ride with him. At first, my fear almost wiped me out, but I started to relax when I accepted that I could trust him to control the bike. He wasn't about to let me fall. Then I realized how freedom really felt! With the breeze in my face, it felt like I was flying! That experience put life in the fast-forward mode for me."

"What is competition like, John?"

John: "It's a combination of trust and power, with a lot of courage thrown in. I have to trust Tom's power. He's got more stamina than anyone I know, and I can always depend on him to give us the winner's edge. I've never felt sorry for Tom because he doesn't feel sorry for himself. I've become a much better cyclist since our partnership developed. He brings out the best in me."

"What is it like for you, Tom? Most sighted people are afraid to ride a bicycle in an arena. How do you explain your success?"

Tom: "Maybe it's because I can't see what's ahead that I can push myself so hard. I have the advantage of never getting demoralized when someone else takes the lead or is gaining on us."

"You must have a complex communications system."

Tom: "Well, I lean my head against John's back for balance, and I've learned to pick up his thoughts and feelings usually before he says anything."

"When is your next competition?"

John: "Since we won the gold medal in the U.S. Finals, we're headed for the world competition next month in Moscow."

"Tom, what would you like to do if you could do anything imaginable?"

Tom: "I'd like to drive a car. In other words, I'd like to be sighted and not be so dependent on people helping me. That won't happen, of course, but you asked!"

"What special talents have you developed to compensate for your blindness?"

Tom: "I've fine-tuned my ability to detect hidden information from a person's voice. For example, Maya, I detect in your voice a higher wisdom from some other dimension. You're an advanced being who is here for some really important reason. I suspected it when I tuned in to your first show. In person, there's no doubt in my mind."

"I am complimented by your observation, Tom. I also believe that my mission is urgent and important. Do you understand how you sensed this?"

Tom: "Pure intuition, from something in your voice. Of course, when you're blind, you're in a semi dream-state or meditation-state. Intuition is much easier to develop when we're not interrupted by visual stimuli. Anyway, Maya, your *Owner's Manual* doesn't need to be revised for the blind. We're your greatest fans. Sight may cause some to not see the obvious. Good luck with your quest, whoever you really are. I know that someday I'll see you, and I mean *really see* you."

"Yes, I believe you. You are special, Tom.

"Thank you, John and Tom, for joining us. Best wishes in Moscow.

"Our next guests are partnership counselors to business and industry. They are departing next week on a lecture tour of China. Please welcome Laurel Golden and Wayne Mosley-Golden."

Wayne: "Hello, Maya!"

Laurel: "Maya, thank you for your inspiring program. You are helping many people to take charge of their lives."

"Thank you, Laurel. How do you train people to

develop trust?"

Laurel: "Our training offers tools to overcome blocks that keep people stuck in nonresourceful behavior. After they release these blocks, they learn to trust themselves and others — the basis of partnership."

Wayne: "Trust is a spiritual state of mind, so part of our training is spiritual in nature."

"Please give us an example."

Laurel: "First I'd like to say that most people have been taught that they live in a fast-paced, high-tech, impersonal world. As a result, many people are completely out of touch with themselves and with nature. We develop layers of defense mechanisms — fear, guilt, resentment, judgment, denial — belief systems that build protective walls around our vulnerable, trusting selves. It's vital to our survival that we reconnect with our Earth home through ceremony and ritual — in that connection we can rediscover ourselves and begin to trust again."

Wayne: "As consultants to a number of high-tech companies, we offer training in partnership and team-building, called Funshops — as opposed to the typical workshop. Recently we offered this training to a group of engineering managers in a beautiful, hot springs, resort setting. When we saw this group, our first thought was, 'How are these left-brained analytics going to cope with our exercises?' Our purpose is to stretch people beyond their comfort level, leading them to greater awareness, both individually and as a team.

"We attribute the success of this Funshop and of all our training to our strong spiritual focus. We began by seating the group in a circle and passing the 'talking stick' — a Native American custom. We decorated a stick with brightly colored ribbon and a feather. It was passed to each participant, who expressed their personal goals for the Funshop. The requirement is that whoever is holding the talking stick is the only one speaking and that person must tell the truth. After some amazingly honest responses, we moved quickly into other exercises that encouraged trust, risk taking, and vulnerability."

"What other types of ceremony and ritual do you use?"

Laurel: "We draw from many native cultures. One of our favorites is a wonderful exercise for releasing blocks such as fear, guilt, judgment — whatever is keeping us stuck. Since our last Funshop was right by a river, it made this exercise very appropriate, but a stream, or creek — any moving water will work. Find a rock on your way to the water, and remember exactly where you found it. Take it to the river, mentally placing your block or fear in the rock, and then put the rock in the running water. Don't choose a rock that is so small that it will wash away. Although if it does, that's okay, too.

"Sit with the rock as the water flows over it, washing away and releasing your particular fear or judgment. When the process feels complete, return the rock to exactly where you found it, honoring it for serving as a vehicle for your growth."

Wayne: "We really stress the importance of returning the rock to its home. That is a way of honoring nature and maintaining harmony by returning things to their proper place."

"What type of responses do you receive to this exercise?"

Wayne: "All the responses have been interesting — most very favorable. For example, one of the managers had expressed a desire to be less judgmental and more vulnerable. That went into the rock, and his feedback during the weekend was that he experienced a new level of trust — of himself and others in the group."

Laurel: "Releasing our blocks is vital to growth, and

this is a gentle form of healing and empowerment.

"Another exercise is excellent for grounding and relief of stress, and again, it involves connecting with nature. Stand next to a tree and visualize luminous roots growing from your feet down into the Earth. See these roots extending deep into the ground, reaching toward the center of the Earth. Feel yourself deeply connected to the ground, immovable because of your strong roots.

"Feedback on this exercise is that it is very calming and opens us up to greater awareness. This exercise, like the previous one, should be done alone, although with practice, you can do this one in your mind at any moment you want to feel more grounded. City-dwellers can either go to a park, or I've known some of our participants who worked with potted trees on their patios! The important thing is that we need to be more balanced — not always in our analytical minds — and this process is part of a return to balance.

"I want to emphasize that if the audience members use the exercises we've been describing, please do so with respect and reverence. They are drawn from the ancient ceremonies and rituals of native peoples and are not to be taken lightly."

"Thank you both for the trust you show by sharing this information. In what other ways do you train people to be more trusting?"

Wayne: "Our favorite exercise takes place during a meal. People work with a partner, and the requirement is that they feed each other, including the beverage. One member of our last group decided that he wasn't very hungry when they were faced with this challenge, but most people find it a memorable experience. The reaction is a good indicator of a person's flexibility and of the ability to accept nurturing. Sometimes the ego — particularly the male ego — gets in the way of allowing ourselves to be nurtured. In fact, our training focuses on partnership, not only with each other, but first of all, with the feminine and masculine energy within ourselves. I recommend this as a fascinating growth experience."

"Tell us about your trip to China."

Laurel: "We've been invited by the Ministry of Education to lead Funshops for school administrators. We'll also be making presentations about our partnership training to top Chinese business leaders."

Wayne: "This trip is a dream become reality — now that personal freedom is becoming globally accepted. With the move by the Chinese government to embrace a free-market economy, it seemed natural that we should be a part of the transformation of their leaders."

"Thank you, Laurel and Wayne, for the work you are doing to return people to partnership and balance."

Audience Member #8: "Your talking about trusting ourselves and gaining awareness has lost me. I feel that I don't even know who I am! Where can I start?"

"Do you mind if I ask you some questions?"

Audience Member #8: "No, go ahead."

"Who are you?"

Audience Member #8: "I just told you — I don't know!"

"Please begin by answering whatever feels right. Who are you?"

Audience Member #8: "Well, okay — I'm a mother. Is that the answer?"

"Thank you. Who are you?"

Audience Member #8: "Again? Okay, I'm a wife."

"Thank you. Who are you?"

Audience Member #8: "I am an attorney."

"Thank you. Who are you?"

Audience Member #8: "I am a successful business person."

"Thank you. Who are you?"
Audience Member #8: "I am persistent."
"Thank you. Who are you?"
Audience Member #8: "I am competitive."
"Thank you. Who are you?"
Audience Member #8: "I am independent."
"Thank you. Who are you?"
Audience Member #8: "I am intelligent."
"Thank you. Who are you?"
Audience Member #8: "I am energetic."
"Thank you. Who are you?"
Audience Member #8: "I am seeking."
"Thank you. Who are you?"
Audience Member #8: "I am loving."
"Thank you. Who are you?"
Audience Member #8: "I am spiritual."
"Thank you. Who are you?"
Audience Member #8: "I am beginning to get it. Thank you."

"In order to know ourselves — trust ourselves and others — it is necessary to become acquainted with our true selves, not our 'act' of all the roles we play in society and in our families. Partnership and trust begin with self-trust and understanding. I recommend continuing this exercise with a partner or use it as a written exercise. If used with a partner, the person asking 'Who are you?' must be totally straight-faced. There should be no response other than 'Thank you.' The exercise should continue for five minutes for each partner. You will discover a depth of self that is open to growth and to partnership."

Audience Member #9: "This trust nonsense sounds real good in a Sunday School class, but I live in the real world. Whenever I've trusted someone, I've always gotten ripped off!"

"Will you give us an example?"

Audience Member #9: "I've got lots of examples. It happens all the time."

"One specific example, please."

Audience Member #9: "Okay. The last time I was on vacation, I paid for a hotel room with an ocean view, plus it was supposed to be a two-bedroom suite. When we got to our room, it was a one-bedroom suite, facing a brick wall. They basically said, 'Take it or leave it.'"

"How did you respond?"

Audience Member #9: "We took the room, but we got even. We took towels and stuff, and I bet we've warned a hundred people about the hotel and the travel agency that booked it."

"Did getting even make you feel better?"

Audience Member #9: "No ... I guess it didn't."

"Do you trust anyone?"

Audience Member #9: "Not really."

"Could it be that your experiences mirror your distrust of others?"

Audience Member #9: "No, I just think people can't be trusted. They're all out to get you!"

"Can you be trusted?"

Audience Member #9: "Uh ... I don't know how to answer that."

"Perhaps that is why you find it difficult to trust others. Imagine what it will be like when you open yourself to trust. Begin by trusting yourself, particularly your intuition. Take the risk of trusting your family, your co-workers, your customers. In addition, trust everything around you — animals, the weather, circumstances.

"In order for everyone to reinforce trust, please take a few moments to relax, close your eyes, and breathe deeply. Allow your mind to take you to your special place — that place where you are perfectly safe and where you experience total peace of mind. Perhaps you are at a beautiful beach, or by a mountain stream. Picture the

beauty of nature surrounding you, hear the sounds, and experience the feeling of total peace of mind.

"Remember a time in your life when you experienced trust. Perhaps you will access a childhood memory of a relative who taught you trust, or you may choose to access the trust you experienced in a personal or professional relationship. If no memory of trust comes to mind, then imagine an experience that you wish had occurred, one involving trust.... Focus on the visual, auditory, and kinesthetic details of the scene, fully associating yourself in this experience of trust.

"Now think of a situation in which you need to be more trusting. Put yourself in the scene, fully trusting yourself and the other person, and see that person fully trusting you. Hear what you both are saying, and experience the feeling of complete trust. Know that this trust is already a reality because your thoughts have created a blueprint for your planned outcome. When you are ready, return your awareness to the present and open your eyes. Repeat this mental imagery at least twice a day until you reach your desired results.

"Will you be courageous enough to continue this process of trust in yourself and others? It will change your world — our world.

"Thank you Rama, Tom and John, Laurel and Wayne, for being our guests. Thank you to our audience for joining us for 'High Performance Adventure.'

"Use your Trust Brainware. When we are trusting of ourselves and others, we can conquer our fears and free ourselves to choose a life of action and fulfillment.

"Please join us next week for an exciting adventure into subconscious understanding. What will it mean to you to be able to control negative self-talk and replace it with life-supporting statements? Our guest will be Dr. Anthony Rogers, a transformational psychologist who will discuss tools that will help you to consciously program your subconscious mind. As a result of using the Subconscious Brainware, your success, as you define it, will be dramatically improved. Our program next week is a vital part of developing your personal Owner's Manual.

"This is Maya Cristal. Remember, a frightened person lives in a frightening world — a trusting person lives in a trusting world."

Announcer: "You may obtain a written transcript of this program and a corresponding Trust Brainware package by calling the number appearing on your television screen."

Chapter 11

The Chamber of Choices

Maya breathed deeply of the crisp fall air. The pungent odor of fallen leaves filled her senses as she completed her warm up and paused to savor the golden autumn afternoon. Radiant aspen trees shimmered against a shocking blue sky, softened by puffs of lazy clouds.

The powerful purr of Rich's emerald green Jaguar broke the silence. Maya watched him smiling self-consciously, as he got out of his car and ambled toward her in obviously new running shoes. Who is this man? she thought. At times he is the stereotype producer — handsome, flashy, and fast-talking. Yet that seems to be an act because there is a gentle, sensitive side — an awareness that shows in the way he looks at me. I wonder who he is.

They began running in the hills near her home, discussing the success of "High Performance Adventure." "You're influencing many lives, Maya. This morning you received hundreds of letters and fax messages. One fax caught my eye. It's in the Jag, but I can give you the general idea."

"I would like that, Rich."

"It was from a woman who said she had exercised her power of choice in a difficult situation at her son's school."

"What happened?"

"She had attended a staffing with her son's third grade teacher, the principal, and the school psychologist. Her son, Toby, had been diagnosed as having attention deficit disorder, and the psychologist wanted to put him on tranquilizers. In fact, so did his teacher and the principal. They basically wanted to turn him into a zombie."

"What did she do?"

"She told them she wasn't comfortable with their diagnosis and that she would take care of the situation. Toby, who belongs to an anti-drug club at his school, said he didn't want to take drugs. So she researched her options and discovered the importance of putting him on a special diet that's free of all food colors and additives. She cleaned out her refrigerator and cabinets, throwing away all the sugar-laden snacks, soft drinks, and everything else that contained dyes or chemicals. That was two weeks ago. She said she can already notice a difference in Toby, and so can his teacher. He doesn't seem 'wired' any more. She was so pleased that she stood up to the system, stating that using her *Owner's Manual* has made her aware of her power of choice in all situations."

"She will enjoy our guests on the 'Healing Adventure' in a few weeks."

"How can you be so calm, Maya? We have received literally thousands of similar success stories, yet you take your phenomenal overnight fame so calmly. How do you do that?"

"I am simply fulfilling my mission, Rich."

Their run had taken them to an area of tall sandstone rock formations, a place of mystical shadows, hidden from the afternoon sun. Maya slowed to a walk, then paused in front of an enormous rock. "Rich, I must stop for a moment." She was staring intently at the rock, when she heard her five tones, gently pulling her into a different dimension. Holding her spirit tones in her awareness, Maya was suddenly traveling rapidly through the rock in a blur of shadows and darkness, stopping at the end of a long tunnel.

She looked around in amazement as her eyes grew accustomed to her surroundings. Reaching out to touch cold, damp stone, she shivered. Why did I choose to come to this place? What am I here to experience?

Gradually Maya became aware of the sound of movement nearby. Peering into the shadows, she saw a figure and said, "Who are you?"

"I am a messenger sent to guide you through the tunnels of darkness to the meeting place."

"Who sent you?"

"That you will know soon. Come, take my hand and follow me."

Maya reached out to grasp a gnarled hand. She felt no fear, only wonderment at her mysterious surroundings. Then the journey began through a maze of tunnels, up and down narrow stairways, led constantly by the nameless guide. Whenever Maya began a question, she was stopped with the same response, "That you will know soon."

They came to an abrupt halt in a low, narrow passage. "Enter the Chamber of Mirrors, Maya. Remember to maintain your awareness." As the guide vanished with silent footsteps, a door at the end of the passage creaked open. An icy blast of wind created an eerie sound, while low moans came from the chamber, followed by the words, "Go away. Save yourself." Maya centered her awareness and stepped forward.

The dimly lit chamber revealed mirrors on each of the walls. Water was spilling down their surfaces like great drops of tears falling onto the stone floor. Vampire bats hung suspended from the ceiling, their menacing teeth glistening in the shadows. Her gaze met that of a young woman, dressed in tattered rags and chained to a rock at the far end of the chamber. "Go away. Save yourself," moaned the woman as Maya approached.

Moving closer, Maya touched one of the chains. At that moment, a large winged creature came whirling toward the woman's face. Maya stepped back as the woman threw herself onto the stone floor, the bat's wings brushing across her back. Maya waited for the next attack. This time, three of the creatures swooped toward the woman who beat them away with her arms, screaming, "Leave me alone, you filthy monsters!"

When the attack ended, Maya questioned, "Why are you here?"

The woman stopped her moaning to whine, "I don't know — life just isn't fair."

"Life as you have ordered it has arrived. Do you not understand that you can leave whenever you choose?"

"Oh, but I don't really stand a chance of getting out of here. Everyone treats me so unfairly," the complaining continued.

"Your chains are not binding you — you are. It is your choice to stay in this place."

"You don't understand. Because you're unafraid, you're protected from harm. You sound just like that old hag that brought you here. She keeps repeating that when I learn to accept responsibility for being in bondage, then I'll be able to choose freedom." She lifted her arms to reveal how loosely the chains bound her. "I can't bear to think of facing those mirrors. I'd rather be in chains than have to face who I really am. Go away. Leave me alone in my misery."

There was another icy blast as the chamber door was opened by the guide. "It is time to move to the bridge, Maya."

As Maya turned to accompany her guide, she gazed at the woman with compassion, stating, "Remember your nobility. Nothing — no one can keep you in bondage without your permission."

Following the guide became less difficult as they climbed to a brightly lit platform surrounded by illumination rods. Below the platform appeared a sea of darkness. "You must step carefully onto the bridge, Maya. It will lead you to the Chamber of Choices. Maintain your awareness as there are grave dangers in crossing this bridge. Except for the most advanced souls, few have had the courage to attempt the crossing."

The guide slipped silently away into the night, leaving Maya staring intently at the first rungs of a rope ladder leading down into total blackness. She tested the ladder, which swayed uncontrollably in the icy wind. After centering her awareness, she did not look back, but stepped confidently onto the rungs and disappeared into the unknown. She moved with quiet assurance, trusting her intuition. The bottom rung of the ladder snapped, leaving her suspended above a dimly visible, narrow, rope bridge.

"Don't jump! That bridge isn't safe." She looked up in surprise at a sour-faced, elf-like being, perched on another ladder nearby and holding a lantern. "No one makes it across that bridge anymore. Can't get anyone to fix it. It isn't safe. Everything's gone to ruin around here. What's the use? Nothing's going to change. You can't make it. I can't make it ..."

His muttering ceased as Maya shouted, "Stop it! Do you not realize how unconscious you are? All your judgment and complaining does nothing. Why do you not repair the bridge yourself?"

"No, no, no, you don't understand. Too much risk. Too many choices. None worth the risk. What to do? What to do?"

Maya shook her head and prepared to jump. Just then, a giant winged creature flew screeching past her, causing her to lose her balance. One foot caught in the ladder, she dangled upside down precariously between the bridge and oblivion. "Jump! Jump," came a quiet message within the screeching of yet more giant bats. Regaining her balance, she released herself into the air, and it seemed for a moment as though she were flying. Then she landed lightly on the rope bridge which greeted her with much creaking and groaning. Reaching out to grab the rope railing, she withdrew her hand in surprise. On the railing was the alive, scaly, writhing body of an enormous snake.

"We are the guardians of the Chamber of Choices," hissed the snake. "What right have you to cross?" As the creature coiled, Maya noticed that there were dozens of slithering reptiles intertwined around the ropes of the bridge.

She focused her awareness on thoughts of respect and acceptance and on her passion to reach her destination. "I must cross. It is my right to choose trust over fear, love over apathy, healing over pain."

The hissing stopped as suddenly as it had begun. Illumination rods burst into light as the snakes moved aside, clearing a natural path across the bridge. The ropes in the middle of the bridge were broken, creating a large gap. Maya swung lightly from one side of the bridge to the other, reaching safety and stepping easily to the lighted platform above her. There the veiled guide was waiting.

"Well done, Maya. You have earned the right to enter the Chamber of Choices."

Harmonic tones emanated from an open doorway.

The guide placed a jewel-encrusted robe around Maya's shoulders, a sweep of magenta bordered in green velvet, adorned with jewels and feathers. She stepped eagerly forward toward a bright light which glowed from a power source hidden deep within the chamber. Many-faceted crystals glittered from the walls of the cave. Even the chamber floor was inlaid with jewels. She walked toward a large chest, overflowing with precious gemstones — diamonds, rubies, emeralds, sapphires, opals, and pearls. As she ran her fingers lightly over their brilliant surfaces, she sensed their energy pulsating through her entire being.

Maya moved deliberately toward an opening at the far end of the chamber, through which she could hear the roar of ocean surf. Just below the cave's opening, crashing waves hurled themselves onto giant rocks. She climbed a narrow stairway, higher and higher, leading to a natural platform surrounded by the rising tide. Her harmonic tones blended with the deafening roar of the surf, creating a healing force that seemed to flow from deep within the Earth.

On the platform stood a tall, regal woman who was vaguely familiar. She looked intently into Maya's eyes, then began to speak. "Welcome, Maya. I am the Galactic Council leader, Tuluma." Her powerful voice rose above the sound of the crashing waves. "Your wisdom and understanding are reflected in the choices that you have made. You have come a great distance in a short time. Do you fully understand the significance of this journey?"

"Yes," Maya replied, recognition flooding her awareness. "Yes, I do understand."

"Your guide has brought you through the tunnels at the center of the Earth. You have come through a place of enormous power, symbolic of the same power which resides within each Earthling."

Maya responded, "For the Earthlings, the idea of

their own power is both frightening and enticing. There are those such as the woman in the Chamber of Mirrors who insist on giving their power away to external forces. They live a life of denial, chaining themselves to their own fears. There are others who are mentally paralyzed by their acceptance of dysfunctional programming. Yet there are many who are willing to release their fears and face the mirror of truth, remembering their true selves and thus transforming their world. These Earthlings value their noble human potential which glows like the jewels in the Chamber of Choices."

"Yes, Maya. Those who walk the Earth filled with doubts and fears have forgotten that deep within them are powerful resources from which they can draw at any moment. Some are apathetic to the point of being without conscious awareness. Teach them with simplicity and with love that the time has come to reassume their personal power as a healing force for themselves and their fragile planet.

"Continue being the mirror of power balanced with love for them to see their true selves, Maya. Urge them to remember their higher purpose as they use their *Owner's Manuals* for positive action."

Δ Δ Δ

Maya turned to find Rich staring at her intently. "Are you all right?" he asked.

"Yes, it is time to return. There is much to be done."

Chapter 12

The Subconscious Adventure

"**G**ood Evening and welcome to 'High Performance Adventure' This is your host, Maya Cristal. Tonight's Brainware package is vital to developing an Owner's Manual for your brain — the 'Subconscious Adventure.' Our guest, Dr. Anthony Rogers, is a transformational psychologist who has recently published a book entitled, **Self-Programming: The Key to Success.** Please welcome Dr. Anthony Rogers."

"Good evening, Maya."

"How do you describe transformational psychology, Anthony?"

"It's a broad field that directs people toward self-empowerment and personal growth. My area of specialization is the power of the subconscious mind."

"Why did you choose this area of specialization?"

"When I was in graduate school, I read a story that changed my life. It was about a railroad yard worker who was responsible for checking freight cars. Late one afternoon, shortly before quitting time, he stepped into a refrigerator car, and the door slammed shut, locking him inside. It was before the days of the emergency latch release inside such cars. He began pounding on the door and screaming for help, but all the other workers had gone home. He realized that he was doomed because the car would not be checked again until the next day. Believing that he would freeze to death, he began writing the physical symptoms he experienced on a piece of scrap paper: 'I'm shivering — I'm getting colder. The numbness is creeping up my legs — I can hardly write ...' The next day, his body was discovered by his co-workers. The police investigation uncovered a startling fact — the temperature in the car was fifty-three degrees! The refrigeration unit had been turned off. Yet the power of the man's subconscious messages was so strong that it caused his death.

"We bring about what we think about. This story helped me realize that our thoughts determine our reality. Since then I've been working with people to change their self-programming, and thus their perception of themselves."

"That is a powerful example. How do you describe self-programming, Anthony?"

"It's programming positive, life-supporting statements into our subconscious mind. Research has shown some rather remarkable changes can occur when we use a few simple techniques that help make our brains more user friendly."

"Please explain."

"Most people have never stopped to examine what their subconscious mind is telling them. Our subconscious accounts for over 90 percent of our body/mind processes. It is as though we have a very expensive computer on our desks, but we haven't bothered to see what kind of software is in the computer's memory or what software programs are available to us.

"Often, when we want to make a change in our lives,

the subconscious mind will replay our dysfunctional programs. This dysfunctional subconscious programming — and most of us have a large share of it — will sabotage our good intentions. For a very simple example, if someone makes a choice to lose weight, they brace themselves for a battle with their hunger, buy tons of low-calorie food, and then, during a moment of weakness, go on an ice cream binge. Their remark might be, 'There I go again. I can't help myself. I just can't stay on a diet.' Their limiting subconscious messages will prove them right.

"We think that comments such as, 'I have no will power' come after the ice cream binge. They do not. The negative program, 'I have no will power' was just sitting there in the subconscious waiting for an opportunity to express itself. The wait is generally a short one."

"What is your recommendation?"

"Based on my extensive work with clients and on personal experience, there is a better way — one that reprograms the subconscious to respond the way we would like. When I first began my doctoral program, I was about fifty pounds overweight and had high cholesterol. I would fight the battle of the bulge for a few weeks and then quit. Soon I would feel guilty, and like a yo-yo, I would start dieting all over again. One day I realized that I had to change my old dysfunctional program by substituting a program that would get results."

"What did you do?"

"My best explanation is to use a computer analogy. Dysfunctional programs in the subconscious are similar to having a computer virus. You never know when the computer virus will strike until it's too late, and the damage has already been done. For example, self-talk viruses can include statements such as, 'There I go again,' or 'I can't help it,' or 'I hate myself when I eat dessert.'

"What I did was similar to installing a virus detector program on a computer. Any time I start self-talk that is self-defeating, I quickly say, 'That's not like me,' or 'I'm really not like that.' I have found this to be an excellent protection against dysfunctional programming. It cleans out our self-talk files if we will use such a statement with persistence and dedication.

"But the next step is vital to taking charge of our subconscious programming. I wrote out a list of positive traits about myself. I started with forty and have built up to over three hundred. Then I made an audio tape of myself repeating each statement three times, with music in a largo tempo playing in the background to accelerate my reprogramming. I call these 'I am' affirmations. Each 'I am' statement is followed by an 'I deserve' statement. For example, 'I, Anthony, am prosperous. I deserve to be prosperous.' Now I have a marvelous, life-supporting tape that I listen to twice a day. As my needs changed — for example, as I lost weight, or as I began my book — I periodically made a new tape, reflecting my progress and new challenges."

"What makes 'I am' statements powerful?"

"It's a matter of attitude and expectations. When we first consciously consider making changes, our attitude says, 'I don't want to.' Next we limit ourselves by saying, 'I can't.' Then we think about the benefits, and we say, 'I might.' After that we move up to thinking, 'I should.' And then we say, 'I want to.' 'I'll try' follows. That indicates desire but does not get us into action. Then we move up the progression to saying, 'I can.' Some people think they are really going to succeed because they are programming, 'I can,' but that only implies having the ability to accomplish something. 'I can' still does not guarantee action. I know someone who went to a motivational meeting and got all filled with hype because the theme was 'You Can Do It.' He went home and covered a coffee can with eyes of famous people from magazine pictures. He called it his 'Eye Can' to remind him that he could be successful. It was a nice idea but didn't motivate him to action.

"Let's take the next step of 'I will.' Now we are beginning to get commitment for the future, but we still are not into action. Think of the answer Moses received in response to his question to God, 'What shall I call you?' The answer came, 'I am.' There is no deeper affirmation of who we really are than to say, 'I am.' Action follows this statement quickly, because at a deep subconscious level, we know we have already arrived at our goal. That is where we must begin — with the acceptance that we've already arrived. All that remains is to manifest what we truly believe we are."

"Tell us more about self-talk, Anthony."

"A friend, who is a psychiatrist, recently told me that he works on self-talk with his patients, above all other areas. He said, 'Who cares what happened years ago? What's important is our perception of an event, how we talk to ourselves about it.'

"I then asked him, 'What is your goal with each patient?' He replied, 'My ultimate goal is to get patients out of treatment as quickly as possible. But that affects cash flow, so ... you know how it goes, we keep them coming back.'

"I was appalled at my friend's attitude but not surprised. Many people are in treatment for years and years, when it is possible for them to take charge of themselves, rather than being in a co-dependent relationship with their therapist. It doesn't have to take a long time to change. In fact the brain/mind is capable of very rapid reprogramming. I once had a client who had been in phobia-cure training for eight months and had only improved by about 50 percent. She met with me for thirty minutes, and through the use of some neuro-associative programming, she has taken control of her life and no longer accesses that phobia."

"Anthony, many audience members are asking themselves, 'Will affirmations work for me?'"

"It is a proven fact that affirmations work. It's simply a matter of which affirmations we use — positive or dysfunctional. For years, I affirmed my weight problem. Therefore, I had a weight problem. Our subconscious accepts everything we say as true. It does not distinguish between truth and fiction. It is our success mechanism that supports whatever we say and expect in our lives. There is a saying, 'We become what we think about.' That is absolutely true. Affirmation statements, especially with frequent repetition, create a blueprint for success. Yet without action, we have nothing happening. It is up to us to add the all-important action step, and then we will create what we have programmed."

"Do affirmations have to be realistic?"

"The way I explain it is that an affirmation should reflect something that we would like to be or have, that is do-able. I have seen phenomenal changes take place when people are willing to accept responsibility for reprogramming their subconscious mind. I have known many people who have drawn to them their ideal job, mate, car, house — you name it! We can make the choice to create our own reality. Again, I want to emphasize that affirmations must be acted upon to work. I am not advocating sitting on a mountain top and meditating all day. We affirm what we want, and then we go to work to create it."

"Where does dysfunctional programming begin?"

"At home, with very young children. What is the first word they learn? 'No!' And it doesn't get any better by the time they go to school. They are basically told to 'Sit down and shut up!' Think of all the limiting phrases we heard as children. 'Don't.' 'You can't.' 'It's going to be tough out there.' 'Don't take risks.' That's a big one. When our parents tell us, 'Be careful — don't get hurt or run over,' they are programming fear into our subconscious. Now, I am not saying that we shouldn't teach children safety. That's not the issue here."

"What a devastating effect this programming has on self-esteem. What can our audience do to correct dysfunctional programming?"

"Develop a strategy to control limiting self-talk — you know that little, nagging inner critic that whispers, 'You can't do that,' 'You should have acted differently,' or 'You're never going to amount to anything!' That inner critic does a fine job of accepting the task of keeping us humble, after our parents, our religious organizations, and the school system have programmed us.

"Whenever you hear yourself saying, 'I should have,' just say, 'Stop!' You can't ever 'should have' done anything. Should have's don't work because we can't go back and replay the past. When we delete the word 'should' from our vocabulary, we will have come a long way toward controlling our dysfunctional self-programming and improving our relationships with others."

"What do you do to silence your inner critic?"

"I have given my critic a name — he's called Buster. My wife calls her critic Gertrude. Just pick a name that seems to fit, and you will find it easier to tell your critic to be quiet. Of course, once we become aware that Buster is nagging at us, we're halfway there. He doesn't like to be exposed. When he gets really out of hand, I imagine loud, raucous, circus music accompanying his whining voice. Another trick is simply to turn down the volume on Buster's voice, and watch him lose his power! Here's another idea. For one week, keep a journal of every time you judge yourself or others. That gives you a handle on when Buster affects you the most. One of my most successful ways to outmaneuver Buster is to yell, out loud, if possible, 'Shut up! Get out of my life!' He will get the message and be less bothersome. At other times, I simply say, 'Yes, I hear you. You are just wanting attention and love.' Then I imagine myself holding Buster in a moment of love and acceptance."

"What happens when people change their dysfunctional programming?"

"By changing dysfunctional programming to positive programming, we radically affect our performance, our success, and our achievement of our goals. Life is our mirror. We draw to us whatever we expect — whatever we believe we deserve.

"Here is a simple story for our audience. A handsome young knight fell in love with his queen, and she with him. They had been seeing each other for a few months, when the king found out about their affair. He became very angry, and being a manipulative gamesman, he told the knight what his fate would be. He placed him in a large arena with a door at either end. He explained that the knight must choose one of the doors. Behind one door were hungry lions ready to devour him. Behind the other door was a beautiful maiden, whose hand he would have in marriage, should he choose that door. The king also explained that the queen knew what was behind both doors. Just before the knight made his choice, he looked at the queen, and she signaled to him which door to choose. Now answer this question. Which door did the queen have him choose: the hungry lions or the beautiful maiden?"

"Anthony, we will pause for a moment so that everyone may select their choice on their consoles.... Thank you. Our studio monitor shows that 80 percent of you chose the lions, 20 percent the maiden.

"I would like to get a response from the audience. Who chose the lions and why?"

Audience member #1: "The queen wasn't about to let another woman have him if she couldn't."

Audience member #2: "I agree. She'd rather see him die than share her true love with another woman."

Audience member #3: "The knight didn't trust the queen, so he chose the opposite door — and the lions gobbled him up."

Anthony: "Wait a minute. This is a fairy tale. You may choose the ending — and you want violence, death in the arena? Who picked the door with the beautiful maiden?"

Audience member #4: "I did. The queen loved him and wanted him to live a happy life. She was above being jealous."

Audience member #5: "I picked the maiden too. I believe in people, so the queen in my story had a loving heart."

Audience member #6: "Stop! Stop! You don't understand. The king was no dummy. There were lions behind both doors. He tricked the queen too!"

"What do these responses represent, Anthony?"

"This is an opportunity to get a very simplistic, but usually quite accurate view of what kind of programming is in our subconscious. We can choose the ending — play God, so to speak — and yet the responses on the studio monitor are 80 percent in favor of a negative outcome. This shows the extent of the dysfunctional programming that runs our lives. Most people believe that we live in a dog-eat-dog, or lion-eat-knight world. In fact, every day we are bombarded with negativity before we even leave our homes. We expose our minds to the news with our morning coffee, and 87 percent of that news is negative. Good news doesn't make headlines. Bad news sells. Some mornings after reading the paper, I no longer have an appetite for breakfast. Then when we get to work, the negativity continues. We are told what is wrong with the economy, what is wrong with management, labor, with us, and what a rough life this is. Even our comic strips depict mostly negative situations, and some of our most popular TV heroes portray boring lives of negativity and underachievement.

"What this negativity is all about is pre-programmed fear. But it doesn't have to be that way. We can release fear and *choose* what we pay attention to. We need to pay less attention to media hype. I'm not suggesting that we ignore what's going on in the world, but one news program a day is enough. Why submerge ourselves in the muddy waters of all the bad news? It's as though we take a bath in muddy water or allow people to dump garbage on our living room floor. If someone came to your house with a bucket of garbage and dumped it on your carpet, what would you say and do? I'm sure you would stop them and make them clean up their mess. Well, most media programming is like a bucket of garbage dumped into our minds on a regular basis. We take better care of our carpets than we do our minds."

"When we develop our Owner's Manuals, we choose how we program our subconscious minds. We are in charge of what determines our reality."

Audience Member #7: "I just can't believe you're saying we should stop watching the news. I'm very proud of being a well-informed individual and wouldn't miss a single opportunity to keep up with what's going on in the world. That's part of being an intelligent human being! What would happen to this nation if everyone took your advice, or if the children grew up ignorant of what was happening in the world? Things would get completely out of control."

Anthony: "Your desire to be informed is commendable, yet it's important to choose wisely from the programs available."

Audience Member #8: "It frightens me to think that

you're saying we should accept your programming as the truth!"

"Please tell us what frightens you."

Audience Member #8: "I don't know — I'll have to think about it — I guess I'm afraid of rebellion."

"Rebellion against what?"

Audience Member #8: "Oh, the church, the state, everything this country stands for."

"Is there something else?"

Audience Member #8: "Maybe loss of control. This subconscious reprogramming stuff is scary. What if you or someone else starts trying to reprogram us? We could all end up losing our freedom!"

"When individuals are concerned about losing their freedom, they are not free. You are constantly bombarded with subconscious programming from others — the media, government, schools, religion. What else do you fear?"

Audience Member #8: "Why do you keep asking me that? I don't know — maybe I'm afraid someone else is going to program my children with things I don't believe in, like all this 'You're in charge' stuff. Then they won't listen to me anymore. They will turn into a couple of hoodlums, rebelling against everything that is good for them."

"You are getting close to understanding. What would happen if they did not listen to you?"

Audience Member #8: "I don't know — maybe they will ignore me, and I'll be all alone."

"Is fear going to stop that from happening?"

Audience Member #8: "I ... I don't know. I'm not sure what you mean."

"Since we attract into our lives the persons and events that match our thoughts and energies, what is your fear going to attract?"

Audience Member #8: "Uh ... more fear?"

"That is correct. If you express fear in your words and actions with your children, they will mirror fear back to you. How could you replace the fear?"

Audience Member #8: "I'm not sure — I really love them. I want the best for them."

"Then teach them love, not fear. When we release fear, we can fill our lives with love. Give your children many positive choices, and trust them. When given a totally free choice, people will choose love. Look into a baby's eyes. There is no fear. Love is natural. Fear must always be programmed."

Audience Member #9: "You can't dump all your dysfunctional programming, can you? I thought your brain retained information forever."

Anthony: "That's a good question. It's a matter of what we pay attention to. The negative will always be there as the other side of the positive. And we don't want to dump all the lessons we've learned — that information remains as our database. But we do choose at every moment where we place our thoughts and energy. For example, if you have a bottle of muddy water, you can cause the water to become more and more clear by pouring in pure, clear water. This will eventually dilute the muddy water. We do the same thing to our dysfunctional programs, by constantly pouring in the positive 'I am' statements which filter out the limiting self-talk."

Audience Member #10: "I recently read Dr. Rogers' book and have started using subconscious programming with my four-year-old son. Instead of reading a bedtime story, we play the 'I am' game every night. He asks me, 'Who am I, Daddy?' I say something like, 'You are confident, Mike.' He responds by saying, 'Yes, I am confident.' He asks me, 'Who am I?' over and over, and I keep giving him positive statements about himself. When the game is finished, he says, 'Is that all?' This kid can't get enough positive programming, and I know it's giving him strong self-esteem. I wish my parents had been able to help me develop an *Owner's Manual* at his age."

"Thank you for your participation.

"It is vital to developing your Owner's Manual that you spend time cleansing your subconscious mind of dysfunctional programming. This mental exercise will help you to do that. Close your eyes and take some deep breaths. Spend a few moments in your special place, allowing yourself to access total peace of mind....

"Visualize a large computer screen in front of you. On it are listed many of the limiting thoughts that you have about yourself. Take a moment to read through the list, adding anything that may be missing.... Now press the delete key on the computer, and watch the entire list disappear. Begin to enter new information — as many of your strengths as you can bring to mind. List these in the form of 'I am' statements. Take your time. There is no hurry. This list is your positive programming....

"Step back and enjoy this list. In the days and weeks to come, you will be able to return to this image and remember your strengths.

"There is one more function you need to perform. Look in the shadows — there is your inner critic observing you. Invite this critic to come closer to read your list. Look carefully at the top of your critic's head, where there is a small valve. Open the valve, and watch all of your critic's power evaporate. Listen to the rush of air as your critic begins to deflate and sag to the floor, finally disappearing through the floor. Now lean back, and enjoy the confident feeling that any time your inner critic begins to act powerful, you can simply open the valve, letting out all the hot air. Relax in the knowledge that you are reprogramming positives to create the reality of your choice. When you are ready, return to this space

and time, and open your eyes.

"Thank you, Anthony, for being our guest tonight, and thank you to our audience members for your participation. When we access our Subconscious Brainware, we discover that we are in charge of our lives and that we can choose to live in a world without fear.

"Next week on the 'Passion Adventure' we will have some fascinating guests. One is a businesswoman who owns her own air freight business. Two others have a passion to share their ideas with people in far-away places of the world. Another guest has written a guide to conscious investing, and we will have two mystery guests. Each will tell you how they are living their lives with passion.

"What will it mean if you chose to live each day, each moment, to its fullest? What if you no longer have to 'go to work,' because you love what you do so passionately that you are living your dream? Next week our program will help you to access your Brainware to live life with passion!

"This is Maya Cristal thanking you for joining us for 'High Performance Adventure.' Remember, life as you have ordered it has arrived!"

Announcer: "You may obtain a written transcript of this program and a corresponding Subconscious Brainware package by calling the number appearing on your television screen."

Chapter 13

Cyruse – The White Wolf

Maya sat in her comfortable chair, stroking Jopie's soft fur. For several days she had sensed that someone, or something was observing her. It was not an uncomfortable feeling. Instead it was an inner knowing, an anticipation. She had been considering several questions in preparation for the next "High Performance Adventure." How can I encourage others to live with passion? How can passion touch apathetic lives? How can I lead others to action?

She began drawing a pair of eyes on a sketchpad. The more she drew, the more alive they became until they seemed to pull her into their hypnotic depths. She continued staring at the eyes, soon entering an alpha state of awareness. The eyes were still there, silently observing her. Allowing her mind to drift, she slipped into a world of misty shadows, announced by five harmonic tones....

Δ Δ Δ

It was a warm summer night. A full moon illuminated Maya's path. She felt a strong desire to reach a large rock formation separated from her by dense, jungle underbrush of vines and waist-high grass.

She heard a rustle in the sea of tall grass ahead. Slowly, irresistibly, she was drawn into the sounds. Adjusting her eyes to the semi-darkness, she began to run toward the unknown. Suddenly she became aware of a form running beside her. She abandoned herself to the inner knowing that guided her, surefooted on the overgrown path. Matching the rhythm of her pace, was her silent companion who took the lead, as they began to climb the hill. The narrow path became rocky and treacherous as it wound higher and higher. One false step could mean a fall of several hundred feet. Yet their pace remained constant as they continued to climb.

Just as they reached the base of the large rock formation, Maya again heard her five harmonic tones and turned to look into the ice-silver eyes that met her gaze.

"Welcome, Maya. I have waited long for you to come to me."

"And I also have been waiting for this moment. I have felt your presence many times, Cyruse."

Her white fur glistening in the moonlight, the powerful creature communicated, "We are one, Maya. Your wisdom and mine are the same — we simply take different forms. I honor the light of understanding within you."

Maya tenderly embraced the white wolf, saying, "I am glad to see you in this dimension, dear friend. We must continue, Cyruse. I sense a strong energy drawing us higher."

The white wolf led the way up the steep path that wound up and around the rock formation. They stopped in a large clearing. "This is sacred ground, Maya, a gathering place for many spirits who are assigned to protect the Earth."

She closed her eyes and felt the harmony within and

around her. Suddenly the entire clearing burst into flames. She touched her cheeks — they were burning from the heat of the fire. "Follow me," said the wolf, as she ventured boldly into the flames. Maya followed without questioning.

As they walked into the center, untouched by the fire, she sensed a familiar presence. There, in a void surrounded by flames, stood her mother, beckoning her forward.

"Come, my daughter. You have arrived at last."

"Mother, I sensed your energy as we were climbing," Maya said as they shared an embrace of love and respect.

"There is great significance to this moment, Maya. We are surrounded by flames, yet they cannot harm us. They represent the fire that burns deep within each Earthling, the fire that many are not aware exists. This flame feeds their burning desire, their passion that enables them to accomplish great tasks. If ignored, the fire remains a mystery that they will fear and never understand how to harness. If abused by greed or hatred, the blaze will consume them. The world is waiting for those who harness this energy, for within these flames is the power to make changes that will save the Living Spaceship Earth.

"Your mission is to fan the flames within the Earthlings so that they will fulfill the vision of a return to balance and harmony."

"How do you recommend that I fan the flames, Mother? Many Earthlings place a high value on maintaining a positive attitude, yet a positive attitude is like a fire that consumes itself. Attitude alone does not bring about change."

"It is passion that compels people to move beyond a positive attitude into action. The *Owner's Manual* is helping to awaken the Earthlings, and your example will challenge them to greater awareness. Farewell, Maya." The image of her mother blurred into a gold-orange glow, then faded completely.

Suddenly, Cyruse lunged through the flames with a deafening howl, leading the way to the safety of the path. As the terrain became more and more steep, Maya noticed huge lava rocks and realized that they were at the edge of an active volcano. Her gaze focused on the orange molten magna glowing far below. Cyruse broke the silence, "The spirits of my ancestors have roamed this land since before it became populated by the Earthlings. Many civilizations have lived in peace and harmony with Mother Earth. Life was a balance of mind, body, and spirit.

"The ancient ways taught that everything is alive — every rock, tree, mountain, river, ocean — the Earth herself — and that we are all relatives who treat each other with love and respect. This changed radically when the invaders — with their black books and firearms — declared their superiority over all other life forms. They have since cleared the forests, restricted movement of all other living beings, and filled the air and water with poisons. Many of the balancing forces have lost not only their homes, but also their noble spirits. Maya, you are our last hope — our only hope for survival. Does the human species have the awareness to recognize that our Living Spaceship Earth must return to balance or die a miserable death, choking on her own waste?"

"Yes, Cyruse. I believe that awareness is returning. There is no alternative."

Cyruse gazed knowingly into her eyes, then leaped toward the molten lava below. Maya stared in shock, followed by relief as the wolf reappeared, soaring like a bird, a stream of fiery sparks trailing her. "Until next time, twin soul," Cyruse communicated. "Remind the

Earthlings that they must take action before it is too late."

Δ Δ Δ

Maya returned to waking consciousness, the watchful eyes urging her to compel her audience to move beyond a positive attitude into passionate action that would assure personal and planetary healing.

Chapter 14

The Passion Adventure

"**G**ood evening and welcome to 'High Performance Adventure.' This is Maya Cristal, your host for the program that involves you in the process of developing an Owner's Manual for your brain. Our first guests this evening represent a total passion and commitment to fulfill their mission. Originally from Holland, they spent twenty years as Christian missionaries in Zaire, giving of themselves in service to others. Please welcome Henry and Claire Leeuwenburg.*"

Henry: "It is indeed an honor to be here, Maya."

"*Thank you. I have been looking forward to having you on our program. Henry and Claire, you have given to others your entire lives. What was your motivation to live in such a selfless manner?*"

Henry: "I think Claire will agree with me. We had a vision, a calling from God to spread His gospel. We just followed that call."

Claire: "Well, Henry, you got the call, and then you proposed, asking me to go to Central Africa with you. I said, 'Yes,' of course!"

"Many would consider you to have extraordinary courage — to go to an unknown land, under unknown circumstances."

Henry: "Well, we had a dream to fulfill. The unknown becomes known when you walk with God."

"You must have had some fascinating adventures."

Henry: "There were many opportunities for adventure. When we first went to Africa, we had to learn the language in three months, adapt to a new culture, a new climate, and deal with the hazards of life in a tropical jungle. Imagine looking at your vegetable garden one morning and seeing a herd of elephants trampling it — or looking into the eyes of a leopard on the front porch of your mud hut — or opening your closet to get a blanket and finding a cobra coiled up in the blanket box."

Claire: "Henry was the one who got to deal with all the snakes. One night during a tropical rainstorm, he was putting on his raincoat, and a snake slithered out of one sleeve. Then when he put his hand on the doorknob, its mate slid to the floor."

"Were you prepared for this life?"

Henry: "No, not really. We tried our best to prepare ourselves, but we didn't know just what to expect."

Claire: "We tried to adjust in advance to doing without modern conveniences, like electricity. We were staying in the capitol, Kinshasa, our first few months. Even though the house where we were staying had electricity, we decided to use kerosene lamps instead, to prepare for life in the interior. We had a servant who didn't know that the house had electricity. In fact, he had just come from the interior, and didn't understand what electric lights were. One day he accidentally discovered the light switch, and came running to get me. 'Look! Look!' he cried in excitement. 'Look at what I can do!' He seemed to think he had created electricity himself. I was so sorry later that we ignored his excitement and immediately turned the lights back off."

"You retired several years ago. Is that correct?"

Henry: "Yes. Although I'm no longer in the full time ministry, I've never considered actually retiring. The day after my official retirement, I accepted the position of part-time pastor for a small church near our home.

"Claire and I are always looking for ways to keep growing. If we don't have a demanding challenge, then we simply work at learning a new language."

"How many languages do you speak?"

Henry: "Altogether, counting three African dialects, ten. The most recent language we learned was Spanish. About five years ago we got some Spanish books and tapes, studied them for three months, and then spent six weeks in Mexico doing mission work. The biggest challenge was being asked to give the morning sermon — in Spanish, of course — by our host, a wonderful Mexican preacher. I only had one hour to prepare, but it worked out well."

"Are you involved in other forms of service?"

Henry: "Yes. We have a prison ministry. We write letters and send Christian books to over two hundred prisoners. In addition, Claire works one day a week as a hospital volunteer, and I serve as a chaplain at the hospital."

"I understand that you both are quite active physically."

Henry: "Yes, people say they can't believe all we do for being in our eighties. I grow a large vegetable garden, and I also keep my horse in the pasture behind our house. I ride her almost daily. In fact, she surprised us with a colt recently, which was quite a thrill.

"Claire rides her exercise bicycle fifteen miles a day, and we both love to walk. I also swim and ride my bicycle quite frequently."

"Do you have other interests?"

Henry: "We both study the piano and practice daily — Claire just recently started taking her first piano lessons. We also do a great deal of reading, and Claire is a published author."

"When were you first published?"

Claire: "When I was eighty-three. I write stories about Africa and also about what it was like growing up in Holland and Belgium. I like people to know we have it pretty good here in America!"

"Henry, you have also published recently, is that correct?"

Henry: "Yes, I have self-published a gospel tract in English, Spanish, and Russian, and am distributing it world-wide."

"What a remarkable life you lead!"

Henry: "Well, we've always believed in being on the go and in doing what we love. Recently, Claire's grand-niece came to visit us from Belgium with the purpose of practicing her English. Unfortunately, all she did was watch TV, with the volume turned off, and read French novels. She completely missed the point of her visit. She certainly didn't have our go-go-go attitude!"

"Tell us about your recent taxi ride."

Henry: "We have a new car, and the electrical system malfunctioned. I had to have it towed and had no way to get to our church the next day, which was Sunday. So I went to the airport to rent a car, and they wouldn't let me rent one because I don't have a major credit card."

Claire: "Henry and I have always paid cash for everything — our car, even our house. So we were shocked when we couldn't rent a car to get to our church."

Henry: "I called a taxi to take us the forty miles. What an unforgettable ride!"

"That is total commitment. I sense in both of you a passion for life — for living with commitment and love. To what do you attribute that?"

Henry: "We've always done what the Lord called us to do. Also, we've been richly blessed by the Lord with each other, with excellent health, and with plenty of opportunities for service."

"Thank you, Henry and Claire, for joining us and for sharing your beautiful story.

"Passion for what you are doing and living a life you feel passionate about comprise the Brainware package that is vital to developing your Owner's Manual."

Audience Member #1: "It sure seems strange to me that you would be endorsing a God-fearing Christian on your program. Most of the troubles in the history of humankind have been caused by religious extremists who knew that theirs was the right cause because God said so. Even within the Christian religion, the Catholics and Protestants of Northern Ireland have been feuding for a hundred years, and they supposedly have the same God. When you get Moslems and Christians together, you can really get a fight going!"

"What are your spiritual beliefs?"

Audience Member #1: "That is not relevant."

"What are your spiritual beliefs?"

Audience Member #1: "Well, okay, I guess you could say I believe in a God who is the God of all religions."

"Are you passionate about your beliefs?"

Audience Member #1: "No, not really."

"Have you been able to make a difference in the world?"

Audience Member #1: "No, probably not, but I feel comfortable with my beliefs and sure don't think people like me will start any wars."

"What we are addressing is the subject of passion, the passion that creates results. Henry and Claire

Leeuwenburg have that passion. What would it take for you to have purposeful passion?"

Audience Member #1: "I guess it would take a cause, a reason for living."

"When you can rediscover a passion for living without needing to have a logical cause, then you will have awakened to life. The Leeuwenburg's love of life is a model of passionate living. They are life. Combine that love of life with a passionate cause, and you will make a difference in the world.

"Our next guest did not play with dolls as a child. Airplanes were her favorite toys. At nineteen she earned her private pilot's license. Her passion for flying led her to train as a commercial pilot while completing college. She later became one of the country's top jet pilots. Today she owns a fleet of jets through her company, Silver Aviation. Please welcome Maggie Silver."

"Hello, Maya. Reverend and Mrs. Leeuwenburg, I enjoyed hearing your story. You certainly exemplify living with passion."

"Maggie, would you agree that you also exemplify the principle of living with passion?"

"Yes, yes, I do. I can remember a discussion I had long ago with a friend. This friend had some health problems and was living in fear. He said he was afraid he would have to live very cautiously the rest of his life — sort of live life halfway. I told him that I would rather live half a life fully than a full life halfway. It has always been my motto to do everything I could — and then some."

"When did you realize that you wanted to be a pilot?"

"I grew up on a farm, so I spent most of my time outdoors. I used to love to lie on the grassy hillside behind our house and watch the birds flying overhead. I knew then that someday I'd be up there with them."

"Have you received discrimination for being a woman

in a male-dominated field?"

"No, I have not received it. It has been there, but I've never allowed anyone else's belief system to affect who I am."

"Who has had the greatest influence on who you are today?"

"That would have to be my mother. She always taught me to believe in myself and to be the best at whatever I did. When I first started school, she told me, 'Do all the assignments the teacher gives you — and then some.' I did just that, and I graduated valedictorian from my high school. Then when I went to college, Mom told me again, 'Do whatever your professors assign — and then some.' I did, and again, had a very good scholastic record.

"When I entered flight school, she gave me the same advice, 'Do everything required by your instructors — and then some.' When I began my flying career, people used to make fun of the hours I would put in — extra training, extra service for our customers, extra paperwork. My peers made fun of me for being so serious. They thought I was crazy! But then I got promoted way ahead of schedule, and my friends quit laughing."

"What motivated you to leave a secure position to found Silver Aviation?"

"I saw ways that I could be more efficient and provide better customer service than anyone around in the air freight industry, so I decided to take the risk and go out on my own."

"You have chosen to make many sacrifices. Has it been worth it?"

"Definitely. I would do it all over again in a heartbeat. Finding your dream and living it is what life is all about."

Audience Member #2: "I'm a wife and the mother of three beautiful children. I can't help but feel sorry for you. I bet you've never known the joys of being a mom."

Maggie: "True, and there's a part of me that does acknowledge that void. But I suppose you could say I've given birth to a successful business that employs a family of workers, plus thousands of young women have told me how much my accomplishments have encouraged them to live a more passionately committed life.

"Let me add that being a wife and mother is no less challenging a life as long as you live with love and passion."

"Thank you, Maggie. Your example is touching many lives.

"Our next guests are an example of living life with extraordinary passion. Author of many books, a painter, and philosopher, this guest and his artist wife are making a surprise appearance. They are Henry Leeuwenburg's brother and sister-in-law, and they have not seen each other in many years. Please welcome Maurice and Janelle Sentier."

Claire: "Oh my! What a surprise, Maurice, Janelle!"

Henry: "It has been ten years since we've seen each other!"

Maurice: "When I found out Henry and Claire were going to be here, Janelle and I jumped on a plane in Peking to be on this program with them."

"Maurice, your life is quite different from your brother's. Yet you are both world travelers and both live life with passion."

Maurice: "Yes, my travels have been more of a personal nature than Henry's, although we do make many contacts around the world that serve as resources for my books and our paintings."

"Would you mind telling us why you chose the last name of Sentier?"

Maurice: "Well, of course, a writer often does that to be more marketable. Also, I chose a name with much personal significance. Sentier in French means path. As a Buddhist, I am constantly studying the path of enlightenment."

"What influenced you to become a Buddhist?"

Janelle: "I'll answer that, Maya. Many years ago, my daughter spent some time in Sri Lanka, and eventually she became a Buddhist. Maurice and I went over there to find out what she was into and decided Buddhism was the path for us, also."

"You must have had some fascinating experiences in your many travels."

Maurice: "When I was much younger, I was a tennis pro and taught tennis to several famous people, including the Prince of Denmark. That was high adventure! I also love sailing and had a sailing vessel built in the style of a Chinese junk. We have sailed halfway around the world on it and have had some marvelous times."

Janelle: "We owned a villa in Belize for many years and because of the location, and our magnificent tennis courts, we attracted some wonderful people who would vacation with us."

"Maurice and Janelle, you have an intensity, a passion for life which emanates from you. To what do you attribute this quality?"

Maurice: "Oh, I suppose we do have a certain amount of 'joie de vivre' you could say, and we do love life with passion. I've always believed in sipping fully from the cup of life, holding nothing back. I suppose both Henry and I got our intensity level from our mother. She was a fighter, a real doer. She had to be."

"And your father?"

Maurice: "He was an alcoholic. Mother divorced him and had to support five of us kids by herself. She had to be tough to survive. Actually, she was more than a survivor — she was a winner!

"I don't see myself as a super-achiever, simply a

lover of life and a contributor to the good of our world. Passion is living at your edges and giving 100 percent. To do less is treason against yourself."

Audience Member #3: "I always thought Buddhists were peaceful people who meditated a lot and just sort of enjoyed the present moment. How can you be a Buddhist and still accomplish so much?"

Maurice: "That is a common misconception. We have found that peaceful acceptance of daily events helps to eliminate fear and worry. In fact, when we fill our lives with peace, then fear, worry, and stress become words we no longer identify with. When you have peace of mind, then passionate living is a given. Of course, some Buddhists choose to live very quiet lives, but they are happy and passionately peaceful. Thanks for your question."

"Thank you, Maurice and Janelle, for being our surprise guests and for giving us a glimpse into your exciting lives.

"Our final guest is a woman whose passion is returning the Planet Earth to a state of ecological balance. Her background is an MBA from Harvard, with fifteen years as an investment counselor with a well-known brokerage firm. She is the author of **Invest in Your Future: A Guide to Environmentally Safe Investing.** *Please welcome Liz Berry."*

"Hello, everyone. Thank you for this program, Maya. You are raising awareness through helping people to develop their *Owner's Manuals.*"

"Thank you, Liz. I believe that is my purpose. How did you develop your passion for the environment?"

"My best friend in college turned me on to this awareness, although I have been an avid recycler since I was a kid. My parents taught me to love and respect the Earth. But Jamie and I used to talk about how we could make a difference. She now has her Ph.D. in environmental engineering and travels all over the world as a consultant to industry."

"Your emphasis is on one of the newer fields."

"Yes, and a growing field. I love money, and I like to help others make lots of it in a conscious way."

"Will you explain that?"

"Well, most investment counselors just go for the biggest bang for your buck, regardless of the ethics of the company involved. For example, the largest corporations have often been the slowest to change. They would rather pay fines for emitting toxic waste into the air and water than to meet new standards. Many of these same companies are still murdering animals for testing purposes and using toxic pesticides. That's not using an *Owner's Manual* for our environment!"

"How does your book help people to make conscious choices?"

"It offers guidelines for evaluating how an investment rates in different categories, including toxic wastes, animal testing, pesticides, their use of sustainable energy rather than fossil fuels, and top management jobs for women and minorities. I even have a blacklist of unconscious companies."

"You cannot be popular with the firms on that list."

"No, I have received some hate mail. But before the book came out, I approached each company and requested to review their action plans to meet environmental standards. Some companies have been very helpful, expressing their desire to make changes, while maintaining their bottom line. Some even asked for help, stating that they knew the environment was a vital issue, but they did not know where to begin to meet new standards in an economically feasible way. I put them in touch with consultants who assist companies with these adjustments."

"Your book will become quickly dated. How often will

you publish an update?"

"We will publish a quarterly supplement and a new edition annually."

"In what other ways are you actively involved in environmental issues?"

"I financially support activist movements that lobby and demonstrate for the environment."

"Have you demonstrated personally?"

"Yes. During college Jamie and I helped to save an old-growth forest in Oregon that was going to be cleared for lumber. We picketed the logging company and finally could only stop the loggers by chaining ourselves to the trees they were going to destroy. There were over two hundred of us involved, and we eventually raised enough money to buy the land and donated it to the state of Oregon as a wilderness area."

"How do you describe passion?"

"It's believing in what you do so strongly that you are 100 percent committed to getting results through action. Putting your beliefs into action really is the key to living with passion. Let me give an example. Many people express concern for the dangers of nuclear waste. Yet do they do anything about this issue? Do they put their money where their mouth is? One of my friends has formed a group called Guardianship of the Earth. She is lobbying to establish sacred sites around all nuclear waste storage areas. Some of these areas have already been declared sacred sites. There is twenty-four hour surveillance by Guardianship of the Earth members. Prayers and meditation are offered twice daily as a reminder of our responsibility to protect our children and grandchildren from a possible holocaust. These sacred sites are needed to remind us of the atrocity of nuclear waste. Those involved in this project are putting their beliefs into action with passion, as are hundreds of other individuals involved in grassroots movements who are working toward a sustainable future for this planet."

Audience Member #4: "I'm the CEO of a major corporation in the building materials industry and a member of a rapidly growing organization that opposes your self-serving views. The only thing I see you accomplishing is book sales for yourself and your publisher. Yesterday we had a group of your 'crazies' picketing our largest warehouse because we still sell redwood lumber. Your people worship those giant trees like they were some sort of ancient God. The majority of our country couldn't care less. When the redwood forests are gone, then we'll use pine or fir, but until then, I say, let the majority rule!"

Liz: "Someday soon your toxic thinking will be just as close to extinction as the redwoods. And you are incorrect — 78 percent of our population is now opposed to harvesting any additional old-growth forests. Ecobalance must start with awareness and self-regulation. Please, let's talk after the program. Reasonable people can surely arrive at reasonable solutions."

Audience Member #5: "Maya, I've really been inspired by your guests, but I've felt enthusiastic about life before. After a few days the hype wore off, and I was back to my normal, dull existence. What can I do to make passionate living a permanent condition, not just hype?"

"When you did feel enthusiasm for life, do you know what caused you to feel that way?"

Audience Member #5: "Nothing in particular. It was just a feeling, a great feeling of aliveness."

"Could you recreate that feeling now?"

Audience Member #5: "I'm not sure ... well, I suppose so."

"Please close your eyes — audience members, please participate in this exercise also. Begin by breathing

deeply to release tension from your body. Picture in your mind a specific time when you had a total passion for living. See the scene, hear the sounds that were occurring at the time, and feel the emotions of that moment....

"Now concentrate on how you were breathing at the time. Relive every aspect of the experience, fully associated in the scene. Play this experience over and over in your mind until you are the very essence of passionate living. Know that you can come back to this state at any time. It is your personal resource. Create what is called a trigger for this state by doing something physical like tapping your collar bone or bringing your thumb and middle finger of your right hand together.

"When you are ready, open your eyes.... I can tell by your reaction that this was a successful experience. My suggestion is simple. Whenever you lose your passion for living, just access this state again and use the same physical trigger. Eventually the trigger will activate the passion — for example, tapping your collar bone will access your experience.

"With passionate action you will be able to bring about personal and planetary transformation, and you can choose to be a part of the solution to the imbalance on the Planet Earth. Apathy has not solved any problems. Passion causes global changes which begin with each individual who takes action. It is your choice. Choose personal freedom for yourself and a future for your children.

"Thank you for joining us, Claire and Henry, Maurice and Janelle, Maggie, Liz, and to our audience.

"Next week our program is entitled the 'Resource Adventure.' Our guest is Dr. Donna Hill, a former Olympic gold medalist, now a consultant to business in the area of human potential and accelerated learning. What would it mean to you if you had a key to unlock your deepest potential, a key to unlock your resources at

the moment when you need them most? Within each of us are amazing, untapped resources that will help us create our lives the way we have always dreamed. Next week you will gain tools which will assist you to access more of your personal power.

"This is Maya Cristal reminding you that life is either a passionate adventure or it is nothing!"

Announcer: "You may obtain a written transcript of this program and a corresponding Passion Brainware package by calling the number appearing on your television screen."

Chapter 15

Thunder Mountain

Maya walked swiftly up the trail to her favorite mountain retreat. She had taken some time to reflect on recent developments in her life. She also needed to be alone in nature. Her Dreamtime experiences had been intensifying, leaving her with a waking awareness of her powers and her mission. Although her memories had not returned completely, Maya remembered a distant home, a Galactic home, and could vaguely picture parents and a brother named Carlos. She knew that she had accepted a mission of great importance which involved bringing an *Owner's Manual* to the 21st Century.

She reflected on the fact that "High Performance Adventure" had become an even greater success than Rich and the network had projected. Maya had never doubted the rapid acceptance of the *Owner's Manual,* but the resistance of certain individuals and religious groups puzzled her. Why would anyone be opposed to personal power and enlightenment, unless they had something to lose by others reclaiming their power. That would explain the death threats she had received. Maya felt compassion for the nonreceptive individuals who were attacking her. Those who feel threatened by the *Owner's Manual* are looking in the mirror of their own fear. She remembered hearing the statement, "Truth has no effect on a closed mind, and it always takes less effort to kill an idea than it does to implement it."

Maya climbed higher and higher, breathing deeply of the clear, cool air. She paused at a rocky ledge overlooking a virgin forest of pine and aspen. The trees below, like graceful dancers, swayed to the rhythm of the gentle breeze. A herd of elk grazed unafraid in a small meadow, while bighorn sheep served as silent sentinels on the granite cliffs a thousand feet above. She would stay here for forty minutes or forty hours or forty days — whatever it took to resolve the questions burning in her mind.

Maya seated herself in the wind-carved arms of a rock throne. Closing her eyes, she began breathing more slowly, entering an alpha state of awareness. She allowed the questions in her mind to float lightly through her awareness. Questions, questions, questions — all answers are simply remembering.

Why would anyone be opposed to personal power and enlightenment? Fear ... fear that is the legacy of organization and control — fear that desires no understanding — fear that is the byproduct of distorted love. Love without understanding begets fear. Understanding without love begets fear. The answer to *Owner's Manual* acceptance is understanding and love. Fear must be diffused by love and followed with conscious understanding.

Are some individuals impossible to reach even with love and understanding? Yes, they have not chosen the path of enlightenment for this moment in time. Old programming is too strong. Perhaps in the next dimension, but not now.

How can *Owner's Manual* information be most effectively communicated to willing individuals? Through simple explanation, examples and open discussion — with understanding, love, and compassion — no time for subtleties.

Can enlightenment always be realized through love and understanding? Yes ... of course. Understanding also implies action. To understand and not act is not to understand.

Maya took a wooden flute from her pocket and began playing her five tones, over and over. Five spirit tones of purest harmony resonated through the forest below, bringing an answering sound of distant thunder. As she reached out her arms to figuratively encompass the mountain, a bolt of lightning was followed closely by a loud rumble of thunder. A few moments later, more lightning and the roar of the wind signaled a mountain storm. She found refuge in the shelter of a small rock formation. The air was charged with electricity, thrilling her with a natural fireworks display. Then the form of Cyruse appeared, untouched by the drenching rain and sleet.

"Unleash the powerful resources within the Earthlings, Maya. It is time for radical change — change that requires passionate truth spoken without possible misunderstanding."

Λ Δ Δ

Safely cradled by the rocks, Maya replayed her Thunder Mountain experience. Then she began her gradual descent, fully energized and with heightened awareness of the urgency of her task.

Chapter 16

The Resource Adventure

"**G**ood evening. This is Maya Cristal, welcoming you to 'High Performance Adventure,' the weekly opportunity to develop an Owner's Manual for your brain. Before I introduce our guest, we have a pertinent question from our audience."

Audience Member #1: "What can you do about a power outage of your brain — at least that's what I call it. Say you've been doing just great using your *Owner's Manual,* and then one day, zap! Your system breaks down because of something unexpected that comes along — some emotional crisis, for example."

"*Thank you for this excellent question. Based on your current Brainware, what steps do you think would be appropriate?*"

Audience Member #1: "Uh, I'm not sure."

Audience Member #2: "I'd like to answer that. First, I'd get by myself where I could concentrate. Then I'd do something that would get my brain functioning so I wouldn't get stuck in my emotions."

"*How would you accomplish that?*"

Audience Member #2: "Oh, I'd go for a walk or do one of the Brainware exercises."

"Thank you for your response. Someone else?"

Audience Member #3: "I recently had the opportunity to test how well the Brainware works under stress. Our company was going through a buy out, and I didn't know if I would still have a job. When the tension got really high at work, I took a short break, went out to my car, and played my 'I am' tape. I sure felt more in charge after that. The key for me is to do something as soon as possible to correct a dysfunctional mental state."

"Thank you for your suggestion. Our Brainware package, Resource States, is a vital tool to deal with these challenging moments. Our guest this evening is a consultant and trainer for numerous Fortune 500 companies, as well as for several Olympic champions. Please welcome Dr. Donna Hill."

"Good evening, everyone."

"Donna, you won an Olympic gold medal in the women's high jump. Is that correct?"

"Yes, that was the summer of 1996. My athletic background has been extremely valuable in my career of training high performers in all walks of life."

"What have you gained from your involvement in sports?"

"I've gained a commitment to myself and others, the discipline of setting an outcome and working to reach it, and a belief in myself and my abilities. Plus, having wonderful friends and being in top physical condition make life more enjoyable. In fact, it's what gave me the idea of developing Resource Training."

"What made you aware of the need for Resource Training?"

"Immediately after completing grad school, I went to work for a national training organization. I was hired to do company profiles and develop training programs. I noticed that some of the companies I worked with had excellent teamwork and communication. They took the time to celebrate victories within their organizations. Even the smallest success was noticed and acknowledged.

"Then there were other organizations that spent a great deal of time dwelling on what was wrong with the economy, with individual departments, or whatever could be used as a scapegoat for their losses. Management ruled their employees by fear and intimidation. Most of these companies are no longer around. They reminded me of what can happen when an athlete gets depressed — lose an event, and they start replaying all their past losses. It becomes a vicious, dysfunctional cycle and is sometimes the cause of their exit from athletic competition. Now the consistent high performers in sports and in business don't give much energy to defeats. They learn the lesson and throw away the experience by refusing to replay a loss over and over in their minds."

"Have you seen a major shift in the focus of training, Donna?"

"Yes. When I first entered this field, we were still using antiquated principles of psychology. For example, behavior modification statements such as, 'Act excited and you will be excited,' are based on the work of William James in the early part of the last century. That's back in the horse and buggy days! This type of psychology takes too much time for today's fast-paced businesses. Also, there's a certain amount of hype and superficiality to 'acting' a way we don't really feel. Trainers and managers using behavior mod are often guilty of false and insincere praise — some call it 'fluff.' Today's business is too sophisticated to have to put on an act. And there are technologies available that far surpass behavior mod in getting rapid, reliable results — methods that honor the integrity of each individual without having people jumping through hoops.

"I might add that dogs are trained by using behavior modification. Dogs lack the ability to rapidly access images, so they need immediate feedback. On the other hand, the human brain can both access and create images. Tapping into our ability to create images greatly accelerates our learning. In addition, the human brain can voluntarily change from a nonresourceful state to a resourceful state. For example, if we get into a state we call depression, we don't have to wait for feedback from someone to change to a state of joy. We can simply access a time when we experienced joy and bring that experience forward to the present moment.

"The difference is between external motivation (behavior mod) and internal motivation (resource states). Resource Training makes us independent of the need for validation from others. We can use our *Owner's Manuals* to access our own powerful resources at any moment."

Audience Member #4: "My question is this — if behavior modification is external motivation and resource states are internal motivation, then it seems as though we are supposed to ignore the comments of others and be totally self-sufficient. That's good theory, but I still love to hear compliments. They really make me feel good. Conversely, an insult does make me feel bad. I guess I'm saying I would still rather have these human emotions than be a 100 percent effective robot. Have I missed the point somewhere?"

Donna: "Psychology is rarely an 'either-or' science. We will never be 100 percent resource state or behavior mod. You simply must choose the technology that serves you best in the moment. For example, my husband is a real charmer. He is constantly telling me he loves me.

He brings me flowers, and we still hold hands at the movies. I love it!

"But occasionally, just occasionally, he will say something harsh to me or perhaps forget a special occasion. At these moments I choose not to get my feelings hurt, but instead I remember the hundreds of times he has been thoughtful and considerate. My grandmother explained it this way. She said, 'You don't have to swallow the bad peanuts' — a crude but effective analogy."

"Donna, how did you develop your Resource Training theory?"

"First, I remembered my own experiences in competition. Just before an event I'd replay all my past victories. These wins became a resource for future wins. I have studied and interviewed high performers in sports and in business, and I found the same thing was true for them. They always drew from their past successes to continue to win big.

"Here's an example. Walter Wilson, last year's Wimbledon Champion, was under a great deal of pressure in his last set for the championship. When reporters asked him what he was feeling during the final intense moments, he said, 'I was thinking about my best matches, my greatest victories. I knew I had the resources to do it again.'"

"You are saying, Donna, that we do not have to 'act as if.' Instead, we can choose to access our own positive resources at any moment."

"Yes, accessing our resource states is very easy. It is something we do naturally all the time, only most people access nonresourceful states far more often than positive states."

"Please give us an example."

"A friend of of mine was explaining how much she had gone through in the process of getting a divorce. As she was complaining, I asked her how many times she had been divorced. She said, 'Just once.' I then asked her how many times she had relived all the painful details. She replied, 'At least a thousand times.'

"'Then you have been divorced 1001 times,' I said, 'because each time you relive the pain, you experience it as if it is happening all over again right now.' I then asked her to remember a wonderful moment in her marriage and to relive that every time she felt hatred toward her ex-husband. She tried it and immediately felt differently toward him. Then she said something profound. 'All this time I've been hating him, it wasn't hurting him — it was hurting me.' She has decided to stop replaying negative events and start drawing from resource states that are going to empower her."

"That is a strong example, Donna. How do you train people to access a positive resource state?"

"I teach them to use VAK understanding from their Communications Brainware, and I'd like our audience to participate in an exercise to demonstrate how this works. Everyone, please stand. First, think of a time when you did something exceptionally well. It could be anything — a promotion, professional recognition, a big sale, a project, something highly creative, a painting or a poem, a sports victory, or a special event such as a graduation. Just pick one experience, and when you've got it in mind, close your eyes and picture every detail around you as if it is happening all over again right now. Be sure to see the experience fully associated, which means from your eyes looking out at the scene.

"Then hear the sounds you heard — what you said, what others said — replaying every auditory memory.

"Next, replay any physical touching, muscle tension, and breathing patterns that occurred during the event. Now feel the feelings you had during this experience. Allow yourself to experience the same emotions over again.

"You will notice a change in your physiology — accessing a resource state gets the adrenalin flowing — your breathing may change, as may your posture and your facial expression. Give the experience you're reliving a word. It could be power, courage, strength, self-confidence, or love — whatever fits for you.

"Visualize a circle drawn on the floor in front of you, a circle large enough for you to stand in. Once you've pictured the circle, give it a color. Choose the first color that comes to mind, and fill the circle with this color. Now go back and relive the experience again. When you have it, take a deep breath, silently saying the word you chose for this experience and stepping forward into your colored circle. Stay in your circle, holding the experience for fifteen to thirty seconds. When you complete this exercise, please be seated."

"I am enjoying your smiles and happy expressions. Who would like to give us your feedback?"

Audience Member #5: "That was great! My circle was red, and my word was power. I went back to when I made my biggest sale ever!"

Audience Member #6: "My color was purple. I was running my first 10 K, and I felt great!"

Audience Member #7: "Mine was self-confidence. I'd done a really good job in making a presentation and got positive feedback from upper management. I picked the color red, also."

Audience Member #8: "All I could see when I closed my eyes was the backs of my eyelids. I just don't get it!"

Donna: "Did you have a concrete example of a past success?"

Audience Member #8: "No, not really."

Donna: "Do you picture things in your mind easily?"

Audience Member #8: "Not at all."

Donna: "Then I want to make two observations. First, don't worry about it. Roughly 10 percent of the population does not visualize easily. They don't remember their dreams very well and usually only remember them in black and white.

"Second, assuming that you would like to enhance your ability to visualize, there are some very simple exercises you can do to strengthen your visual acuity. Maya, these exercises will be in the Brainware package for this week, right?"

"Yes, Donna. It may help to understand that people who do not visualize easily have a heightened kinesthetic or auditory sense. What we recommend is that you intensify the senses that you already have highly developed when you are accessing resource states. It is important to realize that everyone needs to continue to develop sensory acuity in the visual, auditory, and kinesthetic channels."

Audience Member #9: "I've been going through a lot of stuff lately at work and in my personal life. In fact, I got involved in something that I'm not sure how I'm going to get out of. I feel discouraged, too discouraged to even try to get into a circle."

Donna: "What is the fear behind your discouragement?"

Audience Member #9: "I don't know — maybe that people will find out that I'm a fake, that ... I feel that maybe ... maybe they won't like me."

Donna: "If you could choose right now, exactly how you would like to be feeling, what word would you use to describe that feeling?"

Audience Member #9: "Oh, I guess it would have to be peaceful."

Donna: "Now, think of a time when you did feel peaceful, when everything was going your way, or when you felt calm and in charge."

Audience Member #9: "Okay ... I think I've got it."

Donna: "Good. Now see, hear, and feel everything

about that experience. When you're ready, take a deep breath, and step forward, just one small step, into your circle, while you say the word 'peaceful.'"

Audience Member #9: "Wow! That was wonderful! I feel such a relief from all that depression."

Donna: "The choice is yours to make at every moment. Are you going to access a state of depression, anger, or bitterness, or are you going to access a positive resource state — a state of excellence — which will allow you to be your true, powerful self?"

Audience Member #10: "I work with someone who is very negative and judgmental. Do you have additional methods that can help me be more resourceful under pressure?"

Donna: "Yes. The Western world has generally accepted the theory that the center of our being is in our head. Many other cultures have accepted a more centered approach to our being. I would like to lead you through a centering exercise that will make you more physically aware of what is meant by 'being centered.'

"Would everyone in the audience please stand. Now, feel the total weight of your body pushing down on your head. Take a few steps, feeling as though your head weighed two hundred pounds. Next, shift the weight to your shoulders. Your head feels light and relaxed, but your shoulders are heavy, heavy, heavy. Take a few steps back and forth, back and forth.

"Now shift the weight to your chest. Your shoulders and head are comfortable and light, but your chest is weighted heavily. Shift the weight to your stomach. Take a few steps, feeling the difference. Next, shift the weight to your hips and thighs. They are heavy, heavy, heavy. Your upper body is light as a feather.

"Now put the weight in your feet — one hundred pounds per foot. Walk around with your heavy feet. Feel the lightness in the rest of your body.

"Here's a quick demonstration. Sir, please remain standing. Where do you have your awareness right now?"

Audience Member #11: "Let me see — I guess it's back in my head."

Donna: "Notice how easy it is to push him off balance. Now place your weight in the center of your body, around two inches below your navel. This is your physical center of gravity."

Audience Member #11: "Okay, I've got it."

Donna: "Notice how much more stable he was when I tried to push him off balance this time. The point, of course, is that when we are in a stressful situation physically or mentally, we are more balanced when we carry our awareness of our being in the center of our body. Use centering. It might seem awkward at first, but a couple of successful experiences will solve that. Martial arts practitioners have been using this tool for thousands of years. Centering will work equally well in business and in personal relationships.

"Another tool is to breathe from your center whenever you feel threatened. First, you have to be sure that you are breathing from your abdomen. Most people breathe in a very shallow manner, denying the body its full supply of oxygen and weakening their defense against emotional stress. I would like everyone to practice abdominal breathing with me. Sit straight, putting one hand on your abdomen and one hand on your chest. Now take some deep breaths. Look down to see which of your hands moved. For correct breathing, both hands need to move slightly.

"Now take a deep breath through your nose and exhale through your mouth. Take another deep breath, this time exhaling through your mouth and making a sound similar to purring for part of the exhale. Don't exhale all the air. Hold your breath at least five seconds, and then complete the exhale. Let's do this three times. Inhale through your nose — exhale making a sound — then hold the breath longer each time, finally completing the exhale. When we hold the breath in this manner, we are centered and very relaxed. The benefits from this centering breathing will last for around thirty minutes. With some practice, you will be able to do this without making a sound."

Audience Member #12: "Donna, I recently completed one of your workshops through my corporation, and I'd like to point out that this tool really works. I had to make a presentation to a group that contained some extremely hostile people. In the past, I would have been a basket case, disasterizing in advance about how I might not respond well in this potentially volatile situation. Before the presentation began, I did the centering breathing. Everything began in a civil manner. About halfway through my presentation, one of the members of the group raised her hand and asked to speak. She came to the front of the room and began reading a list of complaints against the program I had sponsored. As she was speaking, I concentrated on continuing to breathe from my center. When she sat down, I acknowledged her right to express her opinion, and then I said that I felt no need to defend my program due to its past successes. People came up to me after the meeting and expressed how much they had gained from my presentation and from my personal power under pressure. I have never felt more in charge and resourceful. Thank you for this tool!"

Audience Member #13, angrily: "I am fed up with all this nonsense on the power of the self! In myself I am nothing. All power comes from God on high!"

"Do you mind if I ask you a few questions?"

Audience Member #13: "Well, yes ... I mean, no ... go ahead."

"When you turn the key in your automobile to start your engine, what is the source of the power?"

Audience Member #13: "The battery, of course."

"And where does the battery get its power?"

Audience Member #13: "From the alternator, I guess."

"And where does its power come from?"

Audience Member #13: "Uh, the gasoline, in the engine."

"And where does its power come from?"

Audience Member #13: "Well, uh, it's made from millions of years of organic materials."

"And where does its power come from?"

Audience Member #13: "Uh, I guess … well, it would have to be from the sun."

"And who made the sun?"

Audience Member #13: "God."

"And does God start your car for you each morning?"

Audience Member #13: "No, of course not."

"I suggest that a way to honor your God is for you to operate your brain with power and integrity. Use your Owner's Manual."

Audience Member #14: "I think I understand your point. God gave us a brain, but we have to use it. But I still have a tough time dealing with criticism. Can Resource Brainware help me?"

Donna: "Yes. I'd like to answer your question with the story of a wise old priestess named Colima, who lived in the high mountains of Peru. People came from hundreds of miles to learn from her ageless wisdom. A powerful, but evil chief from the coastal lowlands decided to discredit the priestess and assume her following. He arrived at her sanctuary and soon received an audience with the ancient one. He immediately verbally attacked Colima, calling her a fraud, a cheat, and a false prophet. He threatened to have her beheaded if she didn't stop dispensing her knowledge.

"She responded calmly with the question, 'If a person offers a second person a gift, and the second person refuses to accept that gift, then to whom does the gift belong?'

"'To the giver, of course,' responded the evil chief.

"'Then I refuse to accept your criticism,' she replied. 'The criticism therefore belongs to you.'

"Whenever someone criticizes you, it is your choice to accept that criticism or allow the giver to keep it. Which is more empowering?"

"Thank you, Donna, for that beautiful story. Do you have some final comments?"

"Yes, I do. There's an old story that emphasizes the beauty and power within each of us. A little girl was watching a sculptor as he began working on a fresh block of marble. She soon tired of what seemed to her to be a slow and boring task. A few weeks later, she again visited the sculptor, and to her amazement, a beautiful lion's head was taking shape under his masterful hands. She watched him for a while and then said, 'Did you know that lion was in there all along?'

"Inside each of us is a beautiful creature waiting to be set free, and it's up to us to sculpt our lives as a work of art, by using our *Owner's Manuals* to remember our true selves and our true power."

"Thank you, Donna. You are a powerful example of the effectiveness of resource states.

"In order to practice your Resource Brainware, take a few moments to calm your mind. Breathe deeply, allowing any tension you may be holding to drain from your body. Now go to your special place where you experience total peace of mind. Allow yourself to sink into the peace and calm that is the center of your true self....

"Imagine yourself in a challenging situation in the past, a situation in which you needed to access a power-

ful resource state, but instead you felt out of control or disempowered in some way. See the details clearly, fully associated, hear what was being said, and relive the emotions that accompanied this experience.... Now recreate this same scene, changing your emotions and responses as you access a resource state by mentally stepping into your resource circle. Notice the difference in the response of the other person involved as you access your positive resource state. Notice the difference in your memory of the experience. We can either choose to internalize painful memories, or we can choose to reframe these experiences by rewriting the script.

"Now think of a situation in the near future that will require a resourceful state. Take a few moments to see the scene, fully associated, as you step into your resource circle, saying your word and seeing the color. Experience the emotions of being completely in charge, as you rehearse the situation from a position of total personal power. Play this mental movie several times, knowing that you are creating a blueprint for your success....

"When you are ready, bring your awareness back to the present space and time. Enjoy your wealth of resources as you develop your Owner's Manual.

"Thank you, Donna, for joining us this evening, and thank you to our audience for sharing your ideas. We value your participation and your commitment to develop your Owner's Manual. Use the Resource Brainware to access your personal strengths.

"Next week, we have a powerful program, entitled the 'Outcome Adventure.' Our guests are Earlene Zigler, who has a remarkable story about her victory over a crippling disease, and Dr. Robert Campbell, a psychologist who trains many high performers, helping them to reach their outcomes.

"What will it mean to you to be able to set your outcomes and reach them? Look forward to moving beyond

goal setting to an understanding of tools that will help you transform your dreams into reality!

"This is Maya Cristal, inviting you to join us next week for 'High Performance Adventure.' Remember, your state of mind can be a conscious choice. Choose wisely."

Announcer: "You may obtain a written transcript of this program and a corresponding Resource Brainware package by calling the number appearing on your television screen."

Chapter 17

The Great Awakening

Maya stepped into the natural, hot springs pool, along the bank of the isolated, mountain river. Torrents of water tumbled over huge boulders, spilling into cascading waterfalls nearby. The sounds of the rushing water and the relaxation of the hot, mineral springs led her to a heightened perception of her intense bond with the Earth.

Drifting into alpha awareness, she sensed an ominous warning. Something was terribly wrong. Her harmonic frequency had never sounded harsh and menacing. The tones were the ones that normally heralded her Dreamtime, yet they sounded threatening, warning of impending disaster.

Centering her awareness, Maya listened intently. There it was again — her five tones in a jangled cacophony of sound. Although there may be danger, or an emergency, I must follow my tones. I am prepared to face the unknown. With this thought, she released herself into Dreamtime awareness.

Swirling masses of clouds prevented her from focusing on her screen. She traveled rapidly through time and space, trusting the discordant tones to guide her. Suddenly the clouds cleared, and two young children came into view — a girl and a boy, who appeared to be sister and brother. They were walking on a forest path, hand in hand, as they approached a fork in the road.

"Which way should we go?" they questioned. "Both roads look the same," said the little girl, shaking her blond curls.

"Then let's take that one," responded her brother, pointing to the path on their left. "Father always said the left means logical and rational thinking."

Maya watched intently as the forest path rapidly led the children into a vast wasteland. Giant trees, shriveled by acid rain and blackened by fires, stood as solemn warnings of the danger ahead. Climbing over fallen trees that blocked their path, they gasped at the sight of dead birds beneath the skeletons of trees. Icy cold blasts of wind stirred the ashes into raging fires, emitting noxious gases. Running from the fire, they came to a lake bed that was completely void of fresh water, with decaying fish lining the shore. They clung together in horror as huge sections of the land around them crumbled and disappeared with an anguished roar.

An unfriendly sun rose in the sickly, yellow sky. The children searched for protection from the scorching heat, but there was none. Seeing that the hostile, poisoned land offered them no hope of survival, they held each other and sobbed. Maya shuddered in horror as a shadow passed over her screen. Distorted, spaceship clouds gathered into churning masses of impending disaster. As her screen darkened, the two children and their devastated planet disappeared from sight. Maya caught her breath in anguish, whispering, "This cannot be. This will not be."

Moments later, as her screen filled with glowing light, the two children reappeared at the same fork in the path. This time the little girl chose the path to the right, stating, "Mother said that the right is the path of the heart." She and her brother walked hand in hand down a path thick with the ferns, liana vines, and orchids of a tropical rainforest. Wild mushrooms grew in small patches along the path. The sound of rushing water from a nearby stream accompanied the melodious songs of brightly colored birds. The children began a gentle climb that led into golden sunlight, with a panoramic view of lush valleys, distant mountains, and sheer rock cliffs towering above the eucalyptus forest below. They were reunited with their mother and father in a peaceful village nestled among the cliffs. Maya observed as the sky smiled a double rainbow, and then the scene faded into shades of blue, green, rose, violet, and gold.

She heard her five tones again, in their pure harmony and sensed the presence of Carlos beside her. After a warm greeting, Carlos said, "All of Mayata is rejoicing because your mission is successful in awakening the Earthlings. Mission *Owner's Manual* is influencing many individuals — those that are ready to remember their true powers."

"Yes, Carlos. But there is still much to be done and little time remaining. There are those who choose to remain in darkness and live their lives ruled by fear."

"They are exactly where they want to be, Maya. Their doubts and fears are their path for the present."

"How can I reach them?"

"They must help themselves. Until they are ready to embrace their personal power balanced with love, all you can do is to be the perfect example of love in action."

"I agree in principle, but in my heart, I want all

Earthlings to experience this awakening."

"That is why you were chosen for this mission, my sister. Look at our screens." They recognized the Earth at a great distance, glowing with a warm, golden light.

"Transformation is occurring, Maya. Hold this image vividly in mind. The light we see is the Great Awakening of the Earthlings that is building momentum."

Suddenly a shadow passed over their screens as swiftly moving darkness blanketed the Earth. A lightning bolt flashed, and the image disappeared. "Your task is extremely urgent," Carlos continued. "The path of self-destruction the Earthlings have chosen must be changed before it is too late. The image of glowing light we saw will happen, must happen, so that the children of the future will have a future. But global changes have to occur in order for our friends to save themselves and their fragile planet. The Earthlings must create a new outcome for themselves and their Living Spaceship Earth. My harmony is with you, Maya, as you continue your mission of love in action."

Δ Δ Δ

She returned from her Dreamtime experience with a passionate desire to inspire her audience to create positive outcomes for the future, a future which the *Owner's Manual* would assure.

Chapter 18

The Outcome Adventure

"**G**ood evening. This is Maya Cristal welcoming you to 'High Performance Adventure.' Tonight's Brainware is Outcome Planning — moving you beyond goal setting to a tool that will help you achieve your desired results. Our first guest has a dramatic story to share with us. She recently completed the fifteen kilometer Tulsa Run, and she did so with the aid of crutches and outcome planning. Please welcome Earlene Zigler!"

"Hi, Maya. Wow! This is exciting!"

"*You are certainly a determined high performer, Earlene. Your story has made headlines in many cities. Please share it with us.*"

"Well, just over a year ago, I set an outcome that I would enter and complete the Tulsa Run. At that time I was able to walk without the aid of my crutches for only five minutes at a time."

"*Have you been on crutches most of your life?*"

"Actually, for thirty-five years I was in a wheelchair. I only graduated to crutches about ten years ago. I was thrown by a horse and paralyzed from the waist down when I was six years old. The doctors said I would be in a wheelchair the rest of my life. Well, not me! I wasn't going to accept that."

"What did you do?"

"I had one more surgery that made it possible for me to learn to walk with the aid of crutches."

"How many operations have you had?"

"I've had nine operations and have spent a total of almost a year in hospitals."

"You have extraordinary courage, Earlene."

"Well, I've just used the mind given to me by God to overcome some obstacles. I think we are all blessed with a very strong mind. When faced with a mountain, I find a way to get over the top or tunnel through. I never quit!"

"Was there a turning point in your decision not to be bound to a wheelchair?"

"Oh, yes. My husband left me when my daughter was five. I had no money and no job. I couldn't pay my bills, and they were going to turn off my electricity. I'll never forget that cold winter morning. My daughter was crying, 'What are we going to eat?' I told her that God would take care of us. That afternoon I got a check for five dollars in the mail from a friend. That was enough to buy oatmeal and milk.

"The next day I went to the landlord of my apartment building and told him I wanted a job scrubbing floors. He said, 'You're crazy. You can't do that! You're in a wheelchair!'

"I told him, 'Don't tell me can't. Can't is not in my vocabulary! Cut that mop handle down, and I'm off to work.' That was my first job."

"What a powerful example you are of total commitment! Where do you work now?"

"I'm safety coordinator at a Tulsa manufacturing plant. In ten years I've never missed a day of work."

"What prompted you to enter the Tulsa Run?"

"I had been a spectator for several years to cheer for some of my friends at work. Then one day I decided it was time to stop being a spectator, so I set the outcome that I would do it."

"How did you train?"

"I started walking as much as I could, extending my time without crutches. In May I walked a mile a day as part of a fund-raising drive for Muscular Dystrophy. Also, I do a lot of physical therapy. I only have time for about four hours of sleep a night."

"Very few people in our audience can comprehend the pain you live with, Earlene."

"Well, I'm used to it. I just look at it as an opportunity to let others know they can overcome obstacles, too. Two weeks before the run, my feet started bleeding whenever I'd walk, and my doctor told me, 'You can't do it, Earlene. Give it up.'

"I said, 'Don't tell me can't! Can't is not in my vocabulary!' So I used some Vitamin E on my feet and some other home remedies, and I did it!"

"What was it like to participate in such an event?"

"Oh, it was a thrill! There were almost ten thousand entrants, and my friends came out to support me. The weather made it tougher because it was a constant, cold drizzle. I had to use my crutches for most of the course, but that didn't bother me. My goal was an obsession! What amazed me was the people who kept trying to get me to quit. People would stop and ask if I wanted a ride. One motorcycle cop kept hounding me, saying, 'Why don't you quit, lady? I've got to open up these streets!' I told him, 'Don't tell me quit! Quit is not in my vocabulary!'

"Some of my friends walked with me, and some cheered me on and took pictures. My daughter and her husband and my grandbaby drove over from Kansas City to wait at the finish line. I was the last one to finish — crutches and all! It took me three hours and forty minutes. I will never forget the feeling of crossing that finish line!"

"My congratulations to you, Earlene, for your perseverance, your courage, and your beautiful spirit. What do you have planned next?"

"Well, my next outcome is to be able to walk totally without crutches, and then I want to learn to drive so I can buy a car."

"What an inspiration you are to our audience. You are able to touch many people with your strength and love. Thank you for being on our program.

"Our next guest is a psychologist who has spent nineteen years studying high performers from various occupations He is the author of numerous books on human excellence. Please welcome Dr. Robert Campbell."

"Good evening, Maya. What a moving victory story you shared, Earlene."

"Robert, you undoubtedly have a theory on what makes people high performers."

"Definitely. I believe that it's the obstacles we overcome that make us or break us. Some people with the same obstacles as Earlene would just sit there and give up. Others use the experience of extreme challenge to grow and build a better life for themselves and others.

"There is a marvelous example of a young boy of about eleven, who lived in a ghetto in New York City many years ago. He had suffered from malnutrition and rickets as a small child. The doctors said he would never be able to walk normally. Well, he too, did not know the meaning of 'can't.' His hero was Joe Sam Mason, all-time great running back for the New Orleans Saints. He had Joe Sam's posters all over his room. When he heard that the Saints were going to be playing in New York, he tried to get a ticket and just could not raise the money. So he convinced the gate keeper to let him stand where he could try to catch Joe Sam's attention on the way to the locker room after the team warmed up. When he saw Joe Sam, he called out, 'Hey, Mr. Mason, can I have your autograph?'

"Of course, he agreed, and as Joe Sam turned to leave, the young fellow said, 'Mr. Mason, you're my hero. When I grow up, I'm going to be just like you. I'm going to break all your records!'

"Joe Sam said, 'What's your name, son?'

"'Orville Thompson, sir.' The rest is history. Orville Thompson did become one of the greatest running backs in the history of football, and he broke all but two of Joe Sam Mason's records."

"That is a powerful example, Robert. Why was Orville successful?"

"Orville was fortunate in that he knew what he wanted. So is Earlene. When people have an outcome that burns in their hearts and minds, they give that outcome 100 percent effort and commitment. This intense commitment is referred to as our 'burning desire.' We can set goals all day long, but unless that goal or outcome ranks high on our list of burning desires, we are just dreaming. If it ranks high as our burning desire, we are going to do whatever it takes to reach that outcome.

"Let me give you a simple example of a high-ranking burning desire. When a baby finally takes its first, faltering step, it then has one burning desire and that is to take the next and the next. How long does a baby keep taking steps, falling down, getting back up, and going for it again? She will continue until she succeeds. That's important to remember — 'I will until.' That baby has setbacks — falling down doesn't feel all that good, but she does not get discouraged. Why? Because she 'will until' she learns to walk. Orville did the same thing in reaching his outcome, and so did Earlene. They practiced the principle of 'I will until' and did not let any obstacle stand in the way of reaching their planned outcomes.

"Maya, I would like our audience to determine their responses to the following scenarios. What would you do if you had just received, tax-free, the following amounts of money: ten thousand dollars, fifty thousand dollars, and ten million dollars? Be sure that you have written down what you would do with each of the different amounts....

"Now for the responses. I have asked this question of thousands of people, and most of them pay bills with the first amount. Many take a trip or buy a fancy automobile or help their relatives with the fifty thousand. What they do with the ten million is the key issue. Please answer at your consoles. Would you remain in your present job or career? Let's check our audience responses on the studio monitor. All right, that looks like about the average response I have been getting — 81 percent of you would not remain in your present job or career. Let's get a few individual responses."

Audience Member #1: "Right now, I have a medical practice, and I'm really burned out. I'd give anything to be a ski instructor, so that's what I did with my ten million — I quit my practice and moved to the mountains."

Audience Member #2: "I quit my job, gave a lot of money away to charity, and spent most of my time fishing on the country estate I would buy."

Audience Member #3: "I quit working so that I could do more of what I love to do, and that's creative writing. But my wife looked at my responses and whispered to me, 'You don't need ten million dollars to write — just a ninety-nine cent legal pad and a pen.'"

Robert: "That's an excellent point. Thank you for your responses. This is a good test to find out what ranks high on your list of burning desires. About 80 percent of the people we survey are not working in a field they truly enjoy. What this tells us is that there are many dissatisfied people in the work force."

"What do you suggest people do if they are not in a position to change careers at this time, Robert?"

"Maya, developing their *Owner's Manuals* is precisely what I recommend. That will help them to understand themselves better — to use their brains effectively to improve conditions in the workplace. Of course, the way to improve conditions anywhere is to work on ourselves. If we are unhappy at work, we need to remember that everything in our lives is our mirror. We need to ask ourselves, 'What is this situation mirroring in me? What do I need to learn from this?' When we learn the lesson, then we can make appropriate changes in our lives. If we just change jobs, we end up taking the same problems with us. There's a saying that illustrates this point — 'wherever I go, there I am.'"

"Robert, it will be helpful to our audience if you will explain the difference between a goal and an outcome."

"Outcome is a much more powerful word than goal for several reasons. First, most of us have set many goals that we didn't attain. In fact, there is probably not a person in our audience who has reached every goal they ever set. We know that we need to set goals in order to be successful, but only about 3 percent of the population has life goals in a written form. Second, there is the intimidation of the word 'deadline.' We get the feeling that if we don't cross that line, we're dead, and that is negative motivation for most of us. On the other hand, we always get an outcome, so why not plan the outcome we want to achieve?

"After all, the expression, 'If you don't know where you're going, you might end up somewhere else' is very appropriate. Most of us set our outcomes much like Christopher Columbus did. When he left Spain, he didn't know where he was going. When he reached America, he didn't know where he was. And when he returned home, he didn't know where he had been. It's a shame that most people don't take advantage of the tremendous power that comes from creating a plan to guide their lives."

"How can our audience set their outcomes?"

"Building on the VAK understanding is very important in outcome planning. When we write down our planned outcome, the likelihood of our reaching that outcome is increased by 10 percent. Then for the visual channel, we need to create a picture in our minds of our outcome. This picture should be in great detail, and we should be fully associated — see the scene from our eyes, looking out. When we picture the results we want and expect, our chances of being successful increase by 55 percent. Next for the auditory channel, we need to hear what we will be hearing when we reach our outcome. And finally, for the kinesthetic channel, feel the emotion we will be feeling when we have reached our outcome. If we will do all of this, we are close to 100 percent more likely to achieve our planned outcome than someone who just hopes to reach their mark. I have heard it said that hope keeps suffering in place. We have to do a lot more than hope when it comes to creating our desired results."

"How often should people use mental rehearsal of their outcomes?"

"I recommend spending two, fifteen-minute periods a day to focus on your outcomes. Choose a time when you are relaxed and in a quiet place. It is worth the effort in order to create the life that you want.

"There was a historical study done with Russian athletes. The first of four groups practiced their sport eight hours a day for the length of the study. The second group spent 25 percent of their time, two hours a day, in a dimly lit room, listening to music in a slow, largo beat, mentally practicing their game. They spent six hours in physical practice. The third group divided their time evenly, four hours of mental practice and four hours of physical. The fourth group spent 75 percent of their time — that's six hours a day — in mental rehearsal. They physically practiced only two hours a day."

"What were the results of the study?"

"It was amazing! The fourth group had the greatest increase in their athletic performance! We can add this same turbo power to our outcomes by using mental rehearsal to learn at accelerated levels — then we are using our *Owner's Manuals!"*

"Do outcomes need to be realistic, Robert?"

"Ask Earlene or Orville or any of the countless people who have overcome incredibly difficult obstacles to reach phenomenal outcomes. I don't want to be accused of telling people they can 'walk on water,' so I will say that outcomes should be do-able. I would rather see a person aim too high and miss than aim too low and hit. The most important point after we go through the steps of finding our burning desire and setting our outcomes is to get into action, just as Earlene did. Perhaps a story would illustrate this point. There were four frogs sitting on a log in the middle of a pond, and one of them decided to jump off. How many frogs were left? Let's get answers from our audience."

Audience Member #4: "Three!"

Audience Member #5: "None."

"Will you register your response at your consoles, please.... Our monitor shows that 95 percent of you think there were three frogs left, and 5 percent think there were none. Robert, what is the correct answer?"

Robert: "The real answer is four! Listen again: there were four frogs sitting on a log in the middle of a pond, and one of them *decided* to jump off. The trouble is, that frog only decided — he didn't do anything about his decision. So all the planning in the world will do us absolutely no good, until we take *action!*"

Audience Member #6: "For every victory story, there are probably one hundred stories of failure. Earlene's story is inspirational, but aren't you just giving people false hope?"

Robert: "Your term 'false hope' is intriguing. The word hope indicates possibility, while false indicates not true. It is no wonder that people are constantly sabotaging their own success. We must use language our mind can positively accept. When we plan a do-able outcome, using accelerated learning techniques, then there is only one thing that can stop us — inaction. There is only one person who can cause us to accept inaction — ourselves.

"Imagine Earlene confined to a wheelchair for life. That was a very real possibility. However, Earlene's *will* — not hope — brought about her desired outcomes. How strong is your will? Are you willing to accept less than 100% of your potential for greatness? Your *Owner's Manual* will put you consciously in charge of your success forces."

Audience Member #7: "I work as a supervisor in a factory and hate my job, but I don't know what I really want to do with my life. My mom worked in a factory till she retired. She was always unhappy, but all she ever did was complain. Are you saying I can change this pattern?"

Robert: "Yes, you can change. I suggest you start by erasing the old program of reluctant acceptance of your present position. See yourself at work doing your assigned tasks. Hear the sounds and experience the negative emotions associated with this job. Now slowly change the picture to black and white, quiet the sounds, and decrease the intensity of the emotions. Reduce the picture to the size of a postage stamp and move it behind you until it disappears. Repeat this process four times, speeding up the process each time.

"Next replace the picture with your most desirable

work situation. Fully associate, seeing what is going on around you. Hear the happy sounds of your work. Intensify the color, sound, and emotions. Enjoy your new position. You are a new person. Repeat this process twice daily until you are comfortable with your new image. Do you think you can do this?"

Audience Member #7: "Yes, but you missed one of my main points. I don't know what I want to do with my life. How can I image something unless I know what it is?"

Robert: "That is an excellent question. Approximately 97 percent of our population does not know what they want to do when they grow up. I suggest you spend some time with yourself to ask some introspective questions. For example, 'What do I enjoy doing in my spare time? What would I do if I knew I could not fail? What did I want to be when I was a child? What professions do I most admire?' The answers are within you. It is never too late to decide what your life purpose is. And that is not to say that we cannot have more than one life purpose. Many people have happily changed occupations several times throughout their lives. The main point is never, never, never accept a life that doesn't fit."

Audience Member #8: "If I did what I really wanted to do and was successful, it would scare me to death. Aren't some of us better off just dreaming?"

Robert: "No! No! No! Never! It is much easier to change your fear of success than to accept less than your potential. Simply use the same reframing procedure that we used for our last questioner. Replace fear with acceptance. What would have happened if Helen Keller had not overcome her fear of success, or Earlene, or countless others who have conquered their fears by being willing to take action? How many potentially great lives have not been fully lived due to fear? Fear keeps us from risking, keeps us locked forever in the familiar. When we release fear through developing our

Owner's Manuals, we transform dreams into reality."

"Thank you, Robert. Your passion for this subject is contagious.

"In order to immediately use the Outcome Brainware, will everyone please close your eyes. Take some deep breaths and relax your mind and body. Now allow your mind to float gently to your place of inner calm. In this place you are totally in charge of the movies of your mind.

"Imagine that you are entering a control room for your brain. See the instrument panel, the large computer and screen. Set the dials on your control panel for an outcome that is important to you. Watch your screen as the scene comes into focus. You are looking at the scene of your successful outcome. Adjust the dials of your control panel, making the scene brighter, the colors more vivid. Increase the size of the picture until it fills the entire wall of your control room. Increase the volume of what is being said by you and by those around you. Intensify the emotions that accompany your successful completion of this outcome. Now, associate fully with this outcome by stepping into the picture. Observe the world as it will be from your point of view. Play this scene through several times very rapidly....

"When you are ready, return your awareness to the present space and time, comfortable with the knowledge that your outcome is now a reality. Commit yourself to replaying this scene twice daily in order to accomplish your desired outcome. Use your Outcome Brainware to create your desired results.

"Thank you, Robert and Earlene, for being our guests this evening, and thank you to our audience for your participation.

"Our program next week is entitled the 'Wellness Adventure.' Our guests are Dr. Kenichi Fukasawa, a practitioner of holistic medicine, and Mary Raymond, an *author and lecturer on the subject of total wellness. What will it mean to you to take responsibility for your own wellness, to release your dependence on an antiquated medical model? Look forward to gaining tools that will dramatically influence your health and well-being.*

"This is Maya Cristal, thanking you for joining us for 'High Performance Adventure.' Remember, life as you have ordered it has arrived! Would you like to change your order? Then set your outcomes to create your desired results."

Announcer: "You may obtain a written transcript of this program and a corresponding Outcome Brainware package by calling the number appearing on your television screen."

Chapter 19

The Tree of Understanding

Traveling on her harmonic frequency, Maya entered a hidden valley, nestled between rugged mountain ranges. Jagged peaks surrounded her, and a sparkling brook flowed past her feet. A pair of ravens drifted effortlessly on the air currents, while high above, a golden eagle soared majestically. I could stay here forever, she thought. Part of you is always here, came floating into her mind.

Maya listened intently for the sounds that would transport her deeper into the magical world between realities. Letting herself sink into her harmonic frequency, she began to move rapidly forward through space and time. Faster and faster, she flowed with the crystal tones, coming to a gentle stop beneath a giant tree. It was unlike any tree that she remembered seeing — and yet it seemed vaguely familiar. Fascinated, she examined the tree more closely. On its branches appeared every variety of fruit imaginable — apples, peaches, cherries, oranges, pears, mangos, plums, figs, papayas, bananas, and countless others. Each of them was ripe to perfection, mouth-watering, juicy....

"What kind of tree could this be?" Maya mused aloud, "and what does it represent?"

"Thank you for asking, my friend. I am the Tree of Understanding."

"I have never seen a more magnificent tree!" Maya exclaimed.

"The many varieties of fruit in their perfection represent the fruit of understanding that is ripening all over the Planet Earth. Your message is reaching the Earthlings who have heightened awareness — those who are ready to accept the gift of themselves, and who are willing to develop their *Owner's Manuals*. And by accepting their true selves, they are releasing a healing force that will impact the entire planet."

"Thank you, beautiful Tree of Understanding. People always have had a desire to fulfill their higher purpose. The *Owner's Manual* allows them to facilitate action without uncertainty. In the past, doubt has undermined many dreams. Yet doubt and fear are released when people know how to utilize their brain/minds."

Suddenly the tree's branches started to tremble, as the fruit changed form into thousands of birds, each bursting into its own melody, creating a harmony that drew Maya into its depths. The birds rose, in unison, joining in one song of joy, and then scattered in every direction.

"You could say that understanding has taken wing," chuckled the tree. "Each of these feathered creatures carries a seed which will be planted in fertile ground. The concepts of love and understanding are being spread all over the world."

Maya responded, "The next program will challenge the belief systems of many who adhere strongly to what is called the medical model. These individuals yield blind obedience to whatever diagnosis is dictated by the medical profession. How can I urge the Earthlings to take ownership of their own healing process?"

"It is true, Maya. The medical model is deeply entrenched in the minds of many Earthlings. Yet, you cannot compromise your position. Health is a matter of choice. Guide your audience to take responsibility for their health through understanding that total wellness is the birthright of each individual."

Maya hugged the Tree of Understanding, who spoke to her once more. "There will come a time when I will embrace you in my protective arms. You are the perfect balance of love and power, of feminine and masculine energy, Maya." An ominous wind stirred the branches as the tree continued, "For some, you are too pure — they consider you a threat to their imbalanced lives. They will be unable to gaze into the mirror of your perfection. Be aware that you are not alone on this mission. Farewell, Starchild. We will meet again."

As she looked up through the branches, a movement in the sky caught her attention. The cloudless sky of azure blue was pierced suddenly by an explosion of brilliant light. What appeared to be a galaxy of stars was cascading toward the Earth in a waterfall of color. Maya felt herself being drawn into their brilliance, moving rapidly on her harmonic tones. Waves of rainbow light filled her being as she floated, untouched, through the heat and flames of molten, liquid stars.

Δ Δ Δ

She returned to conscious awareness, retaining a partial recall of her Dreamtime, with glimpses of a beautiful valley and a talking tree that spoke of understanding. And then she heard it again — the birds were singing one song, one verse, a uni-verse. Yes, she thought, the universe is that one song which we all sing in unison.

With the joyful remembrance of other dimensions of reality came the understanding that there could be danger in such awareness. Yet Maya knew she was prepared to face the unknown with power and purpose.

Chapter 20

The Wellness Adventure

"**G**ood evening. This is Maya Cristal welcoming
you to 'High Performance Adventure.' The subject of
tonight's Brainware is the 'Wellness Adventure.' Our first
guest is a physician with fifteen years experience in an
inner city hospital and eleven years in private practice. He
has just published a controversial book, **Death by Diagnosis**. Please welcome Dr. Kenichi Fukasawa."

"Good evening, Maya. What a pleasure to be here!
Please call me Ken. All my clients do."

"Ken, after years of practicing traditional Western
medicine, you have made a dramatic change to a wellness model. Please tell us why you made this transformation."

"I spent the early years of my career diagnosing people who were expecting to be told what was wrong with
them. That's what they paid me for. I witnessed a myriad of examples of stress-related diseases, cases where
people were begging for a diagnosis that would give
them something to really worry about. In the Western,
left-brained model of medicine, doctors study diseases,

not prevention of disease. Actually the word is dis-ease, because it is a sign that we are not at ease with ourselves, our bodies, and our lives.

"Let me tell you a story. Once upon a time there was a woman who had somehow convinced herself that she had a bullfrog in her tummy. She went to her doctor, complaining of terrible stomach pains caused by this imaginary bullfrog. The doctor saw her time after time, assuring her that the problem was all in her head. Finally, he became fed up with her repeated visits and told her he would operate. He administered an anesthetic and sent an assistant to find a bullfrog. When the woman awoke, he showed her the frog, saying that now all her worries were over. Indeed, she had been right about the bullfrog, and he had removed it. She went home, thrilled at having had her problem removed. The next day, her neighbor came over to visit and marvel at her 'miracle' cure. Then her neighbor asked her, 'But what if the frog laid eggs while it was in your stomach?'"

"What a strong example of how the power of suggestion can cause dis-ease."

"Yes, and it is the norm in our so-called modern medical practices today. We encourage people to believe the worst, and they never have a moment's peace of mind. I asked one of my clients — I refuse to use the condescending term 'patient' — if she was ready to give up worry, since it was causing her to have all sorts of problems. Her astonished response was, 'Give up worry? Why, of course not! Worry is necessary. It prepares us for all those bad things that are going to happen to us!'"

*"Ken, your book, **Death by Diagnosis,** is causing quite an uproar in the medical community. Will you explain your thesis to our audience?"*

"This book represents years of research showing

that diagnosis kills people faster than illness. Many doctors are playing God with people's lives. 'You have to do what the doctor tells you' is a threat used to coerce us into cooperating with medication. The medical profession overdiagnoses, overmedicates, overoperates, and overreacts much more often that the innocent patient suspects. Of course, obedience to a higher authority is a symptom of disempowerment of individuals who neglect to take responsibility for their own health. The word 'doctor' is ranked just below God in authority and respect. I insist that my clients call me Ken instead of the more conventional Dr. Fukasawa, in order to remove the barriers between us.

"I have a new client who had been through all kinds of tests and had been doctor-hopping to find someone who would give her a diagnosis she could live with — or perhaps die with. She had convinced herself she had cancer, and after all the test results were in, she received a rather anticlimactic diagnosis of candida. Candida was a fad disease some years ago. If doctors didn't know what else to tell a patient, they handed down the verdict of candida, a type of yeast condition.

"This particular client had been on heavy medication and still was not feeling better. She came to me on a referral and out of desperation. The first question I asked her was, 'How are your symptoms serving you?' She was shocked at my question."

"What was her response?"

"She didn't know how to answer. I explained that I teach my clients to dialogue with their symptoms by asking themselves these two very important questions: 'What do I need to learn from this?' and 'Why did I create this in my life right now?'

"My client then explained some of the stress she had been under. Her twenty-year-old son, Rob, had come home on holiday from an out-of-state university with new spiritual views that challenged the traditional beliefs of his family. He was making statements that his parents traced to his association with a group of friends involved in Eastern philosophy. My client pressed him to admit he was wrong and give up his 'new-found heresy.' The more the parents pushed, the more resistant Rob became, until he flew into a rage and started breaking dishes and things. His parents called the police to take Rob to a mental institution, where he underwent psychiatric testing. My client and her husband were actually disappointed when Rob was not diagnosed as mentally ill. They would have felt better if they could have explained his behavior as some form of personality disorder. My client's symptoms were quite simply a manifestation of the disorder in her family life."

"Are you saying that your client chose this condition?"

"At an unconscious level, yes. Everything in life is always a matter of choice, and our choices are directly related to our belief systems. For example, years ago I worked with another physician who had a terrible cough. I urged him to get an x-ray, and he kept putting it off. One day, he agreed, and the x-rays disclosed that he had lesions on his lungs, which were diagnosed as malignant. Six months later, he was dead. After his death, I discovered that x-rays had been taken two years earlier. The same size lesions showed up but evidently were not noticed by his physician. He died after he was *diagnosed* as having cancer. Belief in the diagnosis kills people more often and more quickly than any illness. Thus, my book is called *Death by Diagnosis*."

"That is a radical statement, coming from within the ranks of the medical profession."

"The only way to awaken people is to state the truth in a dramatic way. My book is filled with examples of people who have suffered and died inhumane deaths, killed by well-meaning but left-brained physicians who are locked into their own limiting belief systems.

"For example, a person is told that she has a 'terminal' illness and that 90 percent of the people with her type of illness are dead within three months. Unless she chooses not to accept the diagnosis, she will fulfill that prophecy and be dead within three months. What kills her? It's a combination of causes. The doctor's negative expectations, mixed with fear, create a feeling of foreboding. Then she receives treatments which totally destroy her immune system. It takes a strong person — spiritually and physically — to survive such a diagnosis.

"Another example is that of a woman in her sixties who was living an active, joyous life. She developed some symptoms and went to the hospital for tests. She was diagnosed as having cancer, and because she belonged to the generation that believed that cancer kills, she died within a year of her diagnosis. When the autopsy was performed, it was discovered that she did not have cancer. There had been a mistake in the diagnosis, a bizarre mix-up of records. Her death was totally unnecessary, another example of *Death by Diagnosis*."

"*Your examples emphasize the absolute necessity of developing an Owner's Manual. When people isolate mind, body, and spirit from their interconnection, the imbalance that is created results in dis-ease.*"

"You are correct, Maya. The interconnection between mind, body, and spirit makes it impossible to simply treat the body's symptoms in isolation. The medical profession must, I repeat, must become holistic, helping the whole person to involve themselves in their own healing process. In fact, rather than using the term disease with my clients, I use 'healing crisis' to describe any time the body is telling us that we need to pay attention to it. Attention is all there is, because we are what we think. What are we paying attention to — disease and illness — or health and wellness?

"Sometimes I assume that the difference between curing and healing is common knowledge, but I had better emphasize it. Curing is getting a quick fix such as taking medication for a backache — or even having surgery. Healing, on the other hand, is a process that releases the cause of the dis-ease, and the individual returns to balance and harmony — physically, and more important, mentally and spiritually. Too many people are anxious to take medication, or undergo surgery, looking for a cure. Their problem may be temporarily relieved, but it will very likely come back in one form or another because they haven't dealt with the cause of the dis-ease.

"My mother — I love her dearly — but she believes everything the doctor tells her. She developed symptoms in one of her legs and spent some time off her feet, using hot packs, all according to the doctor's orders. She was feeling much better the day before her appointment to have her leg re-examined. Then she was given her diagnosis, along with the admonition that it would take a long time for her inflammation to heal, and she returned home temporarily crippled."

"You have shared some dramatic examples, Ken. Perhaps you could give our audience a demonstration of how our minds can affect our bodies."

"Of course, Maya, that would be excellent. Everyone please close your eyes, and picture the tallest building you have ever seen — many, many stories high. Get on the elevator, and go all the way to the top of the building. As you get off the elevator, notice that there is a room with the door open. Go into this room and walk toward the balcony. Now step out onto the balcony, and look down at the material the balcony floor is made of.

Notice if it is concrete, tile, or marble. Listen to the wind as it whips around the corner of the building.

"There is no railing around the balcony. I want you to walk slowly to the edge. Look down for several seconds.... Come back from the edge — crawl if you have to — but come back from where you were standing. Please open your eyes.

"May we get some response from the audience about what they were feeling in their bodies?"

Audience Member #1: "I started panicking when the doctor said there was no railing. My hands started sweating, and my heart felt like it was in my throat!"

Audience Member #2: "I couldn't force myself to look down. I was too scared."

Audience Member #3: "I am deathly afraid of heights. I'm glad there's a doctor in the studio because I nearly passed out."

Audience Member #4: "I forced myself to go near the edge. Then I almost threw up."

Ken: "Why did each of you choose fear? What message was your mind telling your body? This experience caused physical reactions that were as real as if you had actually been on that balcony. The power of the mind to affect our bodies is phenomenal. Whatever we think, we create — and this visualization gave you the opportunity to create what was in your mind.

"Why did you choose to be afraid? One of my clients experienced this visualization and chose to glide down from the balcony on a magic carpet. What a delightful way to handle this challenge!

"Now, so that you can choose a better experience, let's go back to the tall building, to the balcony. Only this time it is going to be different, because you can fly. Please close your eyes again. Walk out on the balcony with confidence. Choose the right moment, flex your feet on the edge of the balcony and jump — now, float down and land someplace beautiful. Open your eyes when you're ready to come back...."

"There is a noticeable difference in the physiology of our audience members."

"Yes, Maya. Although it is common knowledge that the mind affects our physiological responses, many people choose to experience fear and pain rather than peace of mind and wellness. For example, even in this visualization, where we can fly to any place we like, one man responded by choosing to land in Central Park, where he was immediately mugged! We must replace such thoughts of dis-ease!"

"Ken, how can our audience deal with their healing crises?"

"It is important to understand that a healing crisis is not the end of the world. The character for the word crisis in Chinese is 'wei-chi,' which means danger and opportunity. When we undergo a healing crisis, we are at a crossroads. We can choose to experience only the danger and accept the traditional Western diagnosis. Or we can choose to go beyond the danger to accept the opportunity, and look at the crisis as a growth experience.

"A key factor in the healing process is the use of intuition — that of the practitioner and that of the client. I have to listen to my inner knowing, which is what I mean by intuition, so that I can guide my client to a path of wellness. The questions I mentioned earlier, 'What do I need to learn from this?' and 'Why did I create this now?' are excellent ways for the individual to learn from a healing crisis."

"Whom can people trust in the medical profession?"

"That is something I want to be very clear about. There are countless medical professionals who have their hearts in the right place — they are caring, honest, and committed individuals who sincerely want to help their patients get well. It is just that they are caught in the old paradigm — the old set of belief systems that isolates a disease and then searches for its cure. That paradigm badly needs to be updated, to encompass a holistic approach to health care.

"I know of a young couple who were looking for an ob/gyn because they wanted a backup for the home delivery of their baby. They planned to use a midwife, but wanted to have a medical doctor, in case of complications. They interviewed many doctors before they found one who met their standards. The husband wanted to catch the baby, as it was delivered. Most of the doctors were shocked when told this and replied, 'You want to do what?'

"This couple realized the vital importance of the bonding process of the baby with both parents immediately after birth, and they would do whatever it took to have the sort of birthing that they knew was best. Now in their state, midwife delivery is illegal. If something were to happen to the baby delivered by a midwife, the couple could go to jail for manslaughter. They were willing to take that risk in order to avoid the typical, modern medical delivery with anesthesia; bright lights; cold, harsh atmosphere; and little chance for immediate bonding of the baby with the parents. It is a sad commentary on my profession that we consider pregnancy an illness and delivery a medical emergency! What used to be considered nature's greatest miracle has become a dehumanizing experience, especially for a woman."

"What can individuals do who refuse to be a part of this system?"

"First, they should accept responsibility for their own health. Then, they should interview doctors before utilizing their services. In my book, I have a list of suggested questions for the interview, such as, 'What is the relation of the body, mind, and spirit in the healing process? What effect does diet have on health? What is disease? What causes disease? What is the role of intuition in the healing process? What do you think of holistic medicine? Do you teach relaxation techniques? Do you believe visualization techniques can speed the healing process?" The responses you receive to these questions will let you know when you have found the right practitioner for you."

Audience Member #5: "What about the role of heredity in illness? My mother had diabetes, and so do I. My doctor told me it's hereditary, and I was bound to develop it."

Ken: "The medical profession has made a fortune off hereditary diseases. It's the prime example of the victim mind-set. My family is a good example. Every male member of my family died from heart disease by the age of fifty. In fact, the main reason I decided to enter the medical profession was to find a way to break this dysfunctional cycle. I didn't discover my answers until I combined the understanding of traditional Western medicine with the holistic model. The answer is balance. I'm sixty-three and in excellent health. Heart disease does not serve me and is not something I buy into for myself. You can do the same with any disease labeled 'hereditary.'"

Audience Member #6: "This whole discussion seems so unreal to me. Your theory is that each of us is totally in charge of our own health, right?"

Ken: "That is correct."

Audience Member #6: "Then please explain to me how my wife and child were 'in charge' of their deaths. Twenty years ago last May, my wife was in a serious skiing accident in Utah. She had to have an emergency blood transfusion, and the local emergency medical people used improperly tested blood. It was one of those one in a million things, but she contacted AIDS through the transfusion. We didn't know it until a month later, but she was pregnant with our son, Skip. My wife died twelve years ago, and Skip followed her a year later. For God's sake, don't tell me they were in charge of their own health!"

Ken: "Sir, God only knows the answer to your question. I've seen individuals diagnosed as having AIDS go into total remission, but as far as your wife and son being responsible for their disease, I don't know — I can't answer that. But, please don't discard holistic health because of your situation. Health is not a black or white, yes or no science. It is holistic. We don't have all the answers yet, but we're going in the right direction. I wish I had a better response for you."

"Thank you, Ken. I applaud your courageous and outspoken stand.

"Our next guest exemplifies what you refer to as the new paradigm, a woman who has rejected the recommendations of her doctors, who told her that she would not live without their medications and surgical procedures. She is the author of two books on nutrition and a well-known professional speaker. Please welcome Mary Raymond."

"Hello, Maya, Ken."

"Mary, you are also active in dispelling the myths of Western medicine. Please tell us about your experience."

"I'm alive and in marvelous health today because I paid attention to my intuition, my 'inner wisdom,' as Ken calls it. As a child, I was raised to believe in the medical model — always in and out of doctors' offices and hospitals with various symptoms. My family considered me a weakling — frail and susceptible to any and all germs. So I grew up with the expectation that illness was the norm and quickly learned that getting sick was a guaranteed way to get attention.

"This pattern continued into my marriage. Ken

described the role of the mind in health or disease. I can trace every one of my symptoms to a cause or need that was not being satisfied on a subconscious level. For example, I had frequently had trouble with stomach aches — digestion was often difficult. These pains always accompanied a stressful, unpleasant event. At the first sign of any pain, I immediately ran to one specialist after another to have it diagnosed. Finally, one doctor gave me a diagnosis that shocked me into awareness. I had been referred to a proctologist, who examined me and flatly stated that I would become nutritionally deficient and eventually die unless my colon was removed.

"I had already developed the courage to question medical opinion. A few years earlier, one doctor wanted to tuck my kidney under, an operation that dates back to just about the time of Noah, and another wanted to perform a hysterectomy. So the colon threat was the final blow! I decided the medical profession was knife-happy, and wanted to finance their expensive sports cars by remaking my body."

"What did you do?"

"At that time, I was teaching college, and started working with a young woman who was a contestant in the state beauty pageant. As the faculty member in charge of the college pageant, I volunteered to help Janet with her wardrobe, makeup, and talent preparations. We were going to shop for her competition gown and had already driven ten miles from her dorm, when she said, 'We have to go back. I forgot to take my vitamins.'

"I couldn't believe what she had said. Who could be that much of a fanatic about taking vitamins? I began asking questions and started reading books on vitamins and nutrition. Back then, a healthy diet for me was a TV dinner and a soft drink. Janet introduced me to a whole new world of awareness. I read that the typical American diet, with its fast foods and instant meals — that are colored, preserved, and plastic-wrapped — offers little actual nutrition. That was when I began changing my eating habits and taking vitamin supplements. I emptied my kitchen of all the sugar, soft drinks, and preservative-laden snacks and started making choices that have dramatically affected my health."

"You were able to avoid surgery?"

"Absolutely. I've continued my personal study of nutrition and realize that I had spent years feeling like I was in poor health, because I believed everything the medical profession told me. For example, I became dependent on pain killers for any discomfort, which made me totally miss the point that pain is simply a way our bodies are trying to communicate with us. They are telling us that something is out of balance, but most of us have learned to ignore our inner wisdom and cover up the imbalance with some sort of pill."

"Are vitamins considered a type of pill by some people?"

"Yes. My former in-laws used to give me a lot of grief about taking supplements. They accused me of being little more than a drug addict. Of course, taking vitamins can be overdone. More than anything, balance is important, and paying attention — learning to cooperate with our bodies' needs."

"Do you agree with the expression, 'We are what we eat?'"

"No, the expression is backwards — we eat what we are. As long as I continued to give my power away to medical doctors, over-the-counter drugs, and a mind-set that said I was weak, I ate the foods — if you can call them that — that expressed what I was. I can remember how I used to decide which junk cereal to purchase. It was the one that my daughter picked because it had the best prize. My daughter might as well have been pouring milk over the box and eating the cardboard, instead of eating the nutrition-robbed cereal."

"Mary, did you change other aspects of your life?"

"Oh, yes! There have been major changes in my life. I have a much stronger and healthier body now in my forties than in my twenties. I've been running and cycling for several years, plus I'm an avid hiker. I've surrounded myself with positive, loving people, and I'm living my dream. I cannot overemphasize the importance of state of mind in creating a life of wellness."

"Congratulations, Mary, for your leadership in the area of holistic living.

"Ken, what is your opinion of the role of nutrition and exercise in the wellness model?"

"In the wellness model, everything is connected — every activity in our lives is a reflection of who we are. For example, if a person gets a headache, instead of covering up the pain instantly with a painkiller, why not go for a walk, breathe some fresh air, and give the body a chance to heal itself? I work with people who are making the choice to rid their lives of dysfunctional programming and to accept peace of mind. So we examine every aspect of their lives — what they eat, what they think, how they breathe, how much exercise they are getting, their emotions, their relationships, their work environment, and their belief systems. We want to make sure that they are experiencing harmony in their choices — that their actions are beneficial to them.

"Here's an example. One of my clients was going through a painful divorce. One evening she finally got the courage to go to a friend's party. One of the first people to greet her said, 'Oh, my dear, I feel so sorry for what you must be going through. Tell me, did your husband run around on you before he left you?' My client immediately left the party in tears and vowed that she was through socializing because it made her so miserable.

"I questioned her concerning why she was choosing to experience misery, instead of peace of mind. She replied, 'I'm not choosing this — that woman just made me mad!'

"I asked if she would prefer to be experiencing peace of mind. She said, 'Sure!'

"Then I told her to close her eyes and sit in the chair the way she would be sitting if she had peace of mind. She immediately moved to a much more relaxed body posture. I asked her to breathe as she would be breathing if she had peace of mind. Her breathing, which had been shallow and agitated, became slower and more regular. I then had her change her facial expression to the way it would be if she was experiencing peace of mind. Right there in my office, within just a few moments, her whole state of mind changed, and she did experience the peace that had been eluding her."

"Most people are not aware that we can control our state of mind by our thoughts."

"Unfortunately, that is true. Since our thoughts work in harmony with our bodies, doesn't it make sense, then, to fill our minds with thoughts that are loving and peaceful? Since we know that we alone choose what we allow to fill our minds, why do we continue to choose fear, and therefore, disease?"

Audience Member #7: "Doctor Fukasawa, I'm appalled at your lambasting of the medical profession. I trust modern science completely, certainly over a bunch of vitamin-popping, attitude-adjusting quacks. I want to know everything in my doctor's diagnosis. It's my right to have his expert opinion of what's going on in my body. That way, I can be prepared for any surprises. After all, I've always said, 'Expect the worst — that way you won't be disappointed!'"

Ken: "I honor your right to strictly adhere to the medical model because it is the holistic way to always respect another's path. But may I ask you a few questions?"

Audience Member #7: "Sure."

Ken: "Do you generally have three to four colds per year?"

Audience Member #7: "Yes ... yes, I do."

Ken: "Do you take a winter vacation each year?"

Audience Member #7: "Yes."

Ken: "Are you ever sick with a cold during your vacation?"

Audience Member #7: "No, I guess not."

Ken: "Why not?"

Audience Member #7: "I don't know why. I've never thought about it."

Ken: "My theory is that you choose not to be sick unless it serves you somehow. Healthy people are generally having too much fun to be sick. Think about it. Do you ever sneeze when you are making love?"

Audience Member #7: "I'm going to sit down now!"

Audience Member #8: "Doctor, are you recommending that the next time a person takes a bite of a candy bar, they should ask themselves, 'What does this say about me?'"

Ken: "At the risk of over-simplification, I would have to agree. Everything in our lives is a mirror of who we are, and thus what we eat tells us a lot about ourselves. Now I'm not saying that we should constantly be asking, 'What does this mean?' and be looking for hidden meanings in everything we do. I'm also not saying that we should feel guilty if we eat a rich dessert once in awhile. Everything needs to be in balance, and we don't need to become fanatics about our diets. We simply need to exercise good judgment. Being holistic is a way of life — a way of living in harmony with ourselves, with others, and with our planet."

Audience Member #9: "I was diagnosed five years ago as having a 'terminal' illness. I didn't like the treatments that were prescribed by the doctors and decided to seek alternative healing. I've been seeing a wonderful physician who has taught me to use visualization to heal my body. Twice a day, I visualize for about fifteen minutes. I see my body as whole and perfect, and it has become a reality. I'm in total remission and have never felt better. My doctor has also recommended that I use laughter therapy whenever I feel the slightest symptoms, and it does work. I watch videos of comedy movies or just indulge in plenty of laugh attacks. Wellness is now a way of life for me."

Audience Member #10: "Dr. Cristal, I'm a new member of T.H.E.M., The Human Economics Movement. I feel this program is a radical departure from everything that has made our country great. You would have us sitting in the dark, listening to soft music, and contemplating our navel when what we really need is medical cures. If I had cancer, I'd want therapy, not voodoo. You should go back to your books and leave medicine to the experts — the real experts, not some weirdo philosopher who calls himself a doctor!"

"When a person feels the way you do, then the medical model is best for them. Do not feel forced to use these ideas. You might simply go for a brisk walk when you have a headache, instead of a taking a pain reliever. Is that something you would do?"

Audience Member #10: "You sound like Satan trying to tempt me. What you are advocating — all this personal power stuff — is the surface of Satanism. You haven't heard the last of T.H.E.M.!"

Audience Member #11: "Dr. Fukasawa, I'm a businessman whose salary depends on our company making a profit. Couldn't you be making more money as a surgeon than as a medical ... what should I call you ... a psychotherapist?"

Ken: "I call myself a holistic specialist, but you may use any term you feel comfortable with. To answer your question, yes, many doctors live on a fast track and depend on expensive surgical procedures to pay their bills. You would be shocked at the number of totally unnecessary operations that are performed. I have also known hospitals that would not release patients in a timely manner due to profit considerations."

Audience Member #11: "If all doctors accepted your methods, the world would only need about half as many doctors. Isn't that right?"

Ken: "Actually, I would estimate we would only need one third as many! However, let me add one major point. There are times when the medical model is 100 percent correct. For example, plastic surgery following accidents is what I consider miracle medicine. Also, cuts, burns, broken bones, certain viral diseases, blood disorders, cataract surgery, and many other conditions benefit from traditional Western medicine. I am not saying that the holistic approach is *the* answer. It is simply an important piece of the puzzle."

"Thank you, Ken. It is vital that all individuals use their Owner's Manuals in choosing how to cope with a healing crises. We must understand that if we are not in charge of our thoughts, then somebody else will be. If we give up control of our health thoughts, then our health is out of control. Refuse to allow that to happen. Health is a choice, not a mystery. It is time for our world to demystify medicine, and that will happen as individuals reclaim their personal power.

"Now, take a few moments to close your eyes and breathe deeply, letting any tension drain from your body. Allow your mind to take you to the place where you experience total peace of mind. Become gently aware of your

breathing. Follow your breath — in and out — a few times. As you do so, begin to imagine a color surrounding your body, a beautiful blue-green. Allow yourself to sink into this healing color. Begin to breathe in the color, bringing it into your body at the base of your spine. Visualize it traveling up your spine, filling the organs of your body, continuing up to the top of your head.

"Now exhale slowly, bringing the color down the front of your body, filling the remaining organs of your body, and allowing it to travel down your legs and flow out through the bottoms of your feet. Repeat this breathing process. Breathe in from your spine, bringing the cool, healing color to the top of your head. Breathe out, allowing the color to spill down your body, permeating every cell with its healing light. As you continue to breathe, saturate any areas of your body that are painful or have been of concern. Know that you are choosing to fill your body and your mind with healing energy....

"When you are ready, bring your awareness back to the present space and time and open your eyes. Repeat this healing visualization as often as you like, remembering that health and wellness are a matter of choice.

"Thank you, Ken and Mary for joining us, and thank you to our audience for your participation.

"Looking ahead to next week on 'High Performance Adventure,' creativity has been called the highest expression of our true selves. Our guests will be Rhonda Browne, founder of Creativity in Action, Inc.; Dr. Helen Windemere, neuroscientist and artist; and Steve Williams, founder of the Whole School concept. They will guide us through the 'Creativity Adventure' on location in Uniqueland, on the Pacific coast of Mexico. Look forward to gaining some tools which will expand your mind and your appreciation for your creative self.

"Until then, this is Maya Cristal reminding you that your health is your responsibility. Respond wisely!"

Announcer: "You may obtain a written transcript of this program and a corresponding Wellness Brainware package by calling the number appearing on your television screen."

Chapter 21

Galactic Messenger

"**M**aya, I must speak with you."

"Come on, Maya. You don't have time to sign another autograph," Rich said hurriedly. "We'll be late for the meeting with the Board of Directors."

The strange looking little man repeated persistently, "Maya, it is urgent that I speak with you now."

"Yes ... yes, of course. Rich, I will catch up with you. This is important.

"Please come into my office," she said. The stranger followed her, waiting to speak until she had closed the door.

"My name is Josh," he stated. Maya looked into what many would consider an ugly face. His eyes were extremely small, close-set, and piercing blue. He held her eyes in a hypnotic stare. "Tell me what you see."

Maya gazed into the compelling eyes and felt herself being drawn into a sea of blue. "You seem familiar to me, but I do not yet remember why."

"But tell me, what do you see?"

"I see wisdom, truth, understanding, love — all these things and more," Maya replied, remaining centered as she felt herself drawn more deeply into the stranger's eyes.

"Maya, it is time for you to know your own secrets on the Earth plane."

In the next instant, she recognized her harmonic frequency, as she was drawn into a whirlwind that lifted her into another dimension of consciousness. She sensed the spirit of Josh and thought his name. Immediately, he appeared beside her in his Galactic form. "The memory is returning. I have known you in another time and space. "

"I was once your most advanced student in Chichen Itza. Now my role is to serve my teacher. I am known as Galactic Agent Josh, and I am one of those assigned to protect you on the Earth plane."

"From what will you protect me, Josh?"

"From persecution in the form of religious extremism; from old-world terrorists; greedy, power-hungry fanatics; government bureaucrats; the military right; and of course, from the most dangerous threat to the *Owner's Manual* — the status quo. But now, there is something I must show you."

Maya's screen opened to a breathtaking view of rainbow lights, swirling in a dance of color. Waves of light swept over her, engulfing her in their depths. Becoming a ribbon of color, she began whirling at light-speed toward a blue-green planet. Wrapping herself around and around the Planet Earth, she flowed faster and faster, and at the precise moment, dove into the atmosphere, plummeting through oceans of sky, islands of feathery-soft clouds, and finally, through the very surface of the Earth, stopping at the planet's fiery core. There she transformed into the purest of crystals, filled with light and energy.

Lifetimes passed before Maya's screen, as her crystal self gradually intensified its power and beauty, changing with the erosion of the Earth. Her evolution placed her at the summit of a tall mountain. There she sensed the presence of two ancient spirits, engaged in an eternal struggle. The One whose garments were totally white was being shown all manner of treasure and worlds that would be His, if only He would fall down and worship the other spirit, shrouded in darkness. Suddenly, the One in white caught sight of Maya in her crystal form, and reached down to pick up this object of pure light and energy, sparkling in the sunlight with great beauty. As the One in white touched her crystal self, He spoke, "This is Truth in its purest form."

The dark spirit, quickly reached toward her, saying gruffly, "Here, give that to me, and I will organize it for you."

Maya's spirit cried out, "No! It must not happen. Truth that is organized will cause utter destruction." But it was too late....

Eons of time passed, and as Maya sensed her crystal self becoming cloudy and dark, she experienced the pain of tormented souls who suffered a sinner's destiny, crying to be saved. Black clouds hid the world from view, while lightning and fierce storms devastated the land. Through the thick mists, she caught sight of warlords, uttering fierce battle cries, ravaging, plundering, and destroying every living creature in their path — all in the name of their God.

The Earth groaned, and Maya sobbed in agony. Warlords changed into huge steel factories, belching smoke and tanks, bullets and blood. The Earth was stained with misery and greed, and still Maya heard the cries. Louder yet were the sounds of the raping of Mother Earth. Fires ravaged her forests, and what was left, fell to the ax of blind, unconscious greed. Blue skies disappeared, yielding a sickly, yellow fog that coated the land. Millions of voices sobbed their last breath in the agony of starvation, as the parched land surrendered withered crops.

The Earth's fever intensified into giant, shuddering earthquakes. In the continued attempt to return to balance, hot tears flowed from volcanic explosions, while great floods released themselves in heaving sobs. Much of the Earthlings' destruction filled the oceans, glutting them with thick, black slime, destroying all life forms in its path.

Maya shuddered at the horror and pain.... "No! No! No!" she cried. "Galactic Consciousness will not allow this desecration of the Living Spaceship Earth to continue."

Using her Galactic powers, she held in mind a different vision — that of a healed planet. Gradually, her screen transformed from dark to light, as heightened awareness brought about quantum changes on the Planet Earth....

Maya became once again the ribbon of color. As she circled the Earth, fresh, green birth greeted her with a new sound — the sound of one song — all life returned to harmony and balance.

Δ Δ Λ

She returned to conscious awareness, wiping tears of joy from her eyes, as she again sensed the presence of Galactic Agent Josh. "I understand the purpose of our meeting, Josh."

"Maintain your awareness of individuals ruled by hate and fear, Maya, for the *Owner's Manual* threatens their very existence and the existence of their self-serving organizations. Our paths will cross again soon." He looked intently into her eyes — then he was gone.

Chapter 22

The Creativity Adventure

"**G**ood evening. Welcome to 'High Performance Adventure.' This is Maya Cristal, your host for the program that involves you in the process of developing an Owner's Manual for your brain.

"Our program this evening is being broadcast on location from one of the most unique facilities in the world. We are at the international headquarters of Creativity in Action, Inc., overlooking the Pacific Ocean, in the tiny independent country of Uniqueland, located just west of Manzanillo, Mexico. Our first guest is Rhonda Browne, the leader of Creativity in Action.

"Rhonda, thank you for inviting us to Uniqueland. Please tell us your story."

"Thanks, Maya. As a child raised in Boston, I was frequently in trouble for being too inquisitive, as are many children. I was different. I refused to silence my curiosity and even questioned many of the answers given by my parents and teachers. My grades were very poor because I often disagreed with 'the truth.' My mentor was an elderly woman who lived in our neighborhood, who kept telling me, 'find out how everyone else is doing something, and then don't do it that way.'

"My first creative idea that was commercially produced was a radar warning device for automobiles. This radar warned the driver when another vehicle was within a predefined corridor of danger. The corridor expanded or contracted according to speed, darkness, temperature, and road conditions. It has reduced minor accidents by 50 percent. I was eight years old at the time. I would come up with innovative ideas, and my dad's engineering firm would produce the prototype. The most important lesson I learned from Dad was that you have to put your creativity into action. Having a great idea is useless unless you act on it.

"Another invention as a child was clothes and shoes that can be expanded as children grow. My most famous invention won the Creative Idea Award for pre-teens. It was a grocery cart with a clock, a calculator, and a small, digital weight scale in the handle. This invention made me seventy-five thousand dollars in the first year alone, and has been paying royalties ever since. I consider it one of my least creative ideas."

"How did you develop Creativity in Action?"

"After barely graduating from college, I started to gather other creative mavericks into a brain pool to come up with unique solutions to tough problems. We were hired by large companies to solve impossible situations. One of our first big successes was with a New York advertising firm. They were having trouble with their advertising campaigns for children's toys. Advertising was so costly that many of their clients were in financial trouble. Our ideas revolutionized toy advertising. We decided that we needed to make a mental impression on the toy user at least three times a day for twenty-one to forty-five days. How could we do it? Easy. Put the advertising on a specially imprinted children's toilet paper. The paper companies were thrilled to have additional revenues. Kids loved the novelty of their own toilet paper, and the environmentalists were happy because we used recycled paper and soy ink, which made the product 100 percent biodegradable. Find out what your competition is doing, and then don't do it that way!"

"Rhonda, you call yourself the leader of Creativity in Action, not president or chairwoman of the board. Why?"

"We don't have any titles at Creativity in Action — titles restrict creativity. Defining anything tends to restrict it. Our associates are partners in uniqueness. Define them, and they are no longer unique."

"I understand that you offer training classes in creativity."

"Yes, but it's a 'good news, bad news' story. The good news is that most people can be trained to be very creative. The bad news is that about half the people trained end up leaving their companies within a year. They cannot handle the restrictions placed on their ideas. Ideas are like children. They must be nurtured and allowed to grow and mature."

"How do you encourage people to think more creatively?"

"We believe that creativity occurs when two or more unrelated ideas collide. For this reason, we teach people to ask dumb questions, rather than smart ones. Smart questions show off how much we know. Dumb ones such as, 'What if?' and 'Why not?' open up creative thinking. We also encourage people to be open and nonjudgmental toward their ideas."

"Your facility is beautifully designed to follow the natural coastline of your country, Uniqueland. Did you and your staff do the planning and architectural design?"

"Yes, we designed the buildings to complement this tropical paradise. The air conditioning utilizes the cool ocean waters. The electricity is generated from the ocean waves and currents and from the wind. Most of our food comes from the ocean and our greenhouses. Bananas, pineapples, papayas, and citrus fruits are locally grown. We have no waste products. Everything is recycled — everything!"

"How did you obtain your own country?"

"Everyone told me that it was impossible to buy land and declare yourself a free and independent country. When I was vacationing in this area many years ago, I knew this was my Uniqueland. I went to the Mexican government officials, and made my request. They refused, of course, and acted rather insulted. I told them that nothing should be impossible — that we just needed to make it beneficial to all concerned. I asked if their country had any problems that Creativity in Action could solve that would justify our exception.

"They agreed that monetary inflation was ruining their economy. If we could solve their inflation woes, then we could purchase our Uniqueland. We locked ourselves in a room for a week to brainstorm the answer. Our solution was accepted immediately, and within a year, Mexico enjoyed inflation control that has totally changed its position into that of a modern, prosperous country. We suggested that they convert immediately to U.S. currency. This increased trade between the two countries and helped stabilize both economies. As you know, several other foreign countries are now using U.S. standards with excellent results."

"What type of government do you have in Uniqueland?"

"None. We have a central clearing house for auto titles and property registration. But no military, police, jails, or taxes. If people disagree, they usually work it out. Everybody understands that Uniqueland is unique, so we don't have normal problems."

*"What are Creativity in Action and Uniqueland say-
ing to the rest of the world?"*

"Be unique — be creative — period. No compromise
— no obedience to other people's norms. The death of
creativity is over-organization and obedience to rules
and regulations."

*"Thank you, Rhonda, for a fascinating view into Cre-
ativity in Action, and congratulations on your commitment to action.*

*"Our next guest is a leader in the field of brain/mind
research, a neuroscientist at Stanford, author of many
articles and books, as well as a painter and sculptor.
Please welcome Dr. Helen Windemere."*

"Hello again, Maya. This is indeed an honor. I'm
highly impressed with your country, Rhonda. My husband and I are envious! We would love to live in such a
paradise."

Rhonda: "You are welcome to visit any time. As you
can tell by the size of our audience, there are many visi-
tors to Uniqueland."

*"Helen, I am delighted to see you again. Please tell
us about brain lateralization."*

"The best known model of the brain is the left-
brain/right-brain theory that we have two hemispheres
which are responsible for performing specific functions.
In most people, the right hemisphere directs the left
side of the body, and the left hemisphere directs the
right side. Traditionally, a right-handed person tends to
be more left-brained and vice versa."

*"What functions are directed by each brain hemi-
sphere?"*

"Here is a vast oversimplification. The left-brain
generally governs logic, analysis, judgment, and linear
thinking. The right-brain generally governs intuition,
emotions, nonjudgment, and lateral thinking."

"How can this understanding benefit our audience?"

"Although no one is strictly right- or left-brained, we do have a preference for one hemisphere over the other. The goal is to use both sides of the brain — the wholebrain — as much as possible so that we are more balanced."

"Tell us about your artistic side and how it fits into the wholebrain model."

"There is nothing more satisfying than tapping into my creativity. I'm much more expressive of my true self when I can get lost in my art than when I'm performing an intricate experiment. In fact, my husband says I become a different person — the woman he first fell in love with."

"Please describe that woman?"

"Oh, she's fun-loving, intuitive, thoughtful of her family. She's the person who takes vacations to Europe, roaming the art galleries or mellowing out in a sidewalk cafe. My artistic self is more balanced and wholebrained in that she doesn't get impatient or sarcastic with her husband and kids like the neuroscientist does. If I didn't have an understanding of wholebrain functions, my marriage would have ended in divorce."

"What can our audience do to be more wholebrained?"

"I recommend a series of exercises to switch on the wholebrain. Whenever we perform an activity that causes us to cross the midline of the body, we are switching on both hemispheres of the brain. These exercises have been extremely helpful with children who have been called 'learning disabled.' In actuality, to the extent that one of our hemispheres is switched off, we are all learning disabled."

"How are these exercises helpful?"

"Because of high-level stress on the job and often at home, we tend to spend a great deal of time being homolateral — either in our left brain or our right. When we are dealing with details — seeing the little picture, as in accounting and technical fields — then we are functioning primarily from the left hemisphere. On the other hand, someone who is feeling highly emotional — really into their feelings, maybe extreme joy or anger or depression — is functioning from the right hemisphere."

"This must cause a great deal of conflict."

"Absolutely! I'll give you a quick example. You've got a man and a woman, both professionals — one has been dealing with details all day — the other has been involved in performance reviews, an emotionally draining situation. Throughout the day and when they both get home, they need to take steps to switch on their brains, or their relationship will suffer. They will not be able to communicate effectively, because they are coming from different worlds."

"Will you show us one of the exercises to switch on the wholebrain?"

"Yes. Everyone please sit straight, with your feet flat on the floor. Now slap your hands twice on your thighs. Next, clap your hands twice. Now crossing your hands, pinch your nose with your left hand, and your left ear with the right hand. Repeat, slapping thighs, clapping hands, and this time, switch to pinch the right ear with your left hand, while also pinching your nose with your right hand. Repeat this at least ten times. Now comes the fun part! Find a partner, and turn to face them. Go through this exercise again, watching them try to find their nose and ears, and maintain their dignity at the same time! This exercise is fun and very stimulating because when we cross the body's midline, we switch on the wholebrain and thus release stress. Also, the laughter is a great wholebrain activity."

"We will be including more exercises in our Brainware package available to each of you in our live and home audience. Helen, please tell us more about brain research discoveries."

"Going beyond the split-brain model is the holonomic

model of the brain, based on extensive research by some brilliant scientists, who compare the way the brain stores data to the way information is stored in a hologram. This research shows that all information is encoded in every part of the brain, although it is accessed in different ways. When there is damage to the brain, for example due to a stroke, we have found that the brain can reinstate lost functions fairly quickly by re-routing the functions to a different part of the brain.

"For example, I have a client, named Veronica, who suffered a stroke which caused paralysis of a portion of the right side of her body and an almost total loss of speech. Yet she has recovered normal speech and in almost every way returned to normal brain functioning.

"The most important part of Veronica's recovery was where she placed her attention and focus. She refused to listen to anyone who said, 'You poor dear. How in the world will you manage?' — as an invalid, they meant. She had the support of her family and a few friends who encouraged her to pay attention to what she could do — paint, work in the garden, and run certain programs on her computer."

"What actions did she take to speed her recovery?"

"She spent an hour a day, sometimes more, using visualization techniques. She also kept a life-sized drawing of a brain in front of her, and visualized her speech center being re-routed to an undamaged part of her brain. She imagined new brain cells learning to perform the tasks that were temporarily out of order. It was a simple process. Her brain naturally cooperated with her body's desire to heal itself.

"The holonomic model of the brain is based on the belief that the brain is an open system — a wholemind which supports life functions, growth, health, and happiness. We can learn a great deal from this theory. Our challenge is to be open to changing our perspective, to transforming any system that is closed — from our limiting belief systems to the way we interact with our environment. An open system doesn't pretend to have all the answers in a neatly packaged formula. Instead, it is open to constant growth and change."

"Thank you, Helen, for giving us a glimpse into the fascinating process of brain/mind understanding.

"Our next guest is an educator, author, parent, and pioneer in the field of alternate-choice learning for children. Founder of the Whole School concept, please welcome Steve Williams."

"Hi, Maya, Helen, Rhonda! Thank you for this wonderful opportunity. Wow! I'd love to bring some of our kids here on a field trip!"

Rhonda: "Consider it done. Talk to me after the show, and we'll make the arrangements."

"Steve, your innovative learning systems have made you a leader in the field of holistic education. Please tell us about Whole School."

"It's a brainchild I had in graduate school. Right now, it's funded as part of the Northern California public school system, but it's only available as a K-5 program. We are adding another grade level each year in order to stay within our funds, and so that the children who started with us will never have to undergo the dehumanizing experience of the old public school system. We take children when they're still very impressionable, and we surround them with a positive, nurturing environment that honors the integrity of each child as a whole person and treats that child with respect and understanding."

"How is this accomplished?"

"Our learning experiences are based on the premise of Plato — that all wisdom is remembering. We treat the children as unique individuals who intrinsically understand what they need to know at a deep, subconscious level. We provide the acceptance and the learning environment for optimum growth and remembering."

"Do you still teach the basics?"

"In a non-traditional way. The old model of public education was based on a left-brained, rational, analytical model. Children were taught to parrot back the correct answer instead of learning how to think for themselves. The fallacy of the old model is that we don't live in a one-answer world. The aim of learning should be far more than merely the accumulation of knowledge. I prefer to use the word 'learning' over the word 'education' because learning is a life-long process."

"You have had some bitter experiences with the old public school system, Steve."

"I think most people have. Many classrooms, not all, but many, were simply assembly line, professional babysitting services, where children were inoculated against thinking for themselves and against, God forbid, daring to be creative!"

"Yet there have been some phenomenal teachers in the old system."

"Yes, we all have been blessed with one or two. Yet one or two caring individuals, no matter how inspiring, cannot hold back the tide of negative conditioning most children experience during their most formative years. There was a research study done recently that followed two-year-olds around over a twelve-hour period. During this time period, the research team discovered that the children were told 'no' by their parents twelve times to every 'yes.' The same study was done with secondary school students, and they received eighteen times as much negative feedback from their teachers as positive. Negative input of that magnitude has had a devastating effect on our youngsters' self-esteem and creativity."

"How is Whole School different?"

"We balance left-brain information with right-brain

experiences, which accelerates learning and makes it fun. Kids should love being in school, and ours do! Our planned outcome is to encourage optimum development of the whole person, honoring differences and cultural backgrounds, in a relationship that is based on trust.

"We have a partnership with the children and their parents to build a strong base of holistic learning experiences. In fact, we think of our school as a business, and it is run that way. The parents and the children are our customers, and without them we wouldn't be in business."

"What kind of holistic learning experiences do you provide?"

"Well, we are constantly innovating, designing methods to encourage strong self-esteem. One of the ways we do this is by teaching centering and the switching on exercises that Helen described — exercises that balance both the left and the right brain. In fact, we begin each day with these exercises, and the kids love them because switching on involves body movement. Our brains switch off rapidly when we are not using movement to keep us from getting locked into a left-brained, strictly analytical type of thinking. We can think better and relate to others more effectively when we switch on our whole brain.

"Another holistic learning experience involves integrating music and art into the learning of math and science. For example, kids create a short musical composition — every room has a piano — or draw or paint or even dance their answers to math and science puzzles. We don't call them problems, by the way. Our kids are constantly encouraged to be creative — to draw, compose, and think outside the lines."

"What kind of test results have the children shown?"

"I deplore having to use standardized testing because it is a left-brain exercise in futility, but we are still testing to maintain our funding. Our test results show an average 17% increase in basic skills over the norm for others in their same grade.

"I want to mention that one of the most powerful tools we use to build self-esteem and avoid performance anxiety is teaching the children to use resource states. When the children access a time when they did something really well, they can anchor that experience as a tool for doing well in some other area such as reading or taking tests. Of course resource state association works with every age. One of our teachers was tutoring her friend, a young executive who was taking a graduate-level math class. His performance anxiety caused him to freeze up on his first exam and get a failing grade of forty. So she worked with him for about five minutes to access a positive resource state. He studied the same way for his second exam as he had for his first. In addition, he accessed his positive resource state and used mental rehearsal. On this exam he got a ninety-five!

"The tools of resource states and mental rehearsal are powerful ways we can provide youngsters with self-empowerment."

Audience Member #1: "What do you do about discipline problems?"

Steve: "My first response to that type of question is that we never allow a child to be labeled as a 'discipline problem.' Having such a label causes a child to misbehave in a manner that lives up to his reputation. Also, we feel that misbehaving is a response to a negative, stressful environment. It is a cry for help. Another cause is that kids simply like to move around all the time — they have a lot of energy. When confined to their desks and told to 'Sit down and shut up,' they respond by wiggling in their seats and acting out. Our children can choose to sit at a desk, or on the floor, or they can stand on the table, if they want to learn that way. We are constantly encouraging them to explore new behaviors, as long as that behavior does not harm them or someone else."

Audience Member #1: "What if their behavior is harming someone, for example, if one child hits another?"

Steve: "Although it seldom happens, such an occurrence is the ideal time to reinforce the conflict resolution skills we teach. We get the children involved to communicate with each other and have them explore different options besides violence. We refuse to act as disciplinarians because that does not encourage self-responsible behavior.

"Sometimes the children get overly excited. We had a good example of that last year. There had been an early snow, and the kids were all excited — yet we couldn't spend the whole day playing outside. We do an exercise we call Japanese breathing, which involves getting everyone seated and breathing in unison with their eyes closed. This continues for a couple of minutes, and the results are remarkable. What the exercise accomplishes is a state of rapport among the members of the group and an openness to learning. This is the way many Japanese companies begin their business meetings, and it works beautifully with all ages. We use this exercise often to open the mind to creative learning."

"Steve, how urgent is it that we stop suppressing the creative abilities in our children?"

"It is vital to their being able to adapt in a rapidly changing world. In fact we are living in a time of great need for innovation in every aspect of our lives. For example, in the business world, if a company does not constantly innovate, does not develop new methods or products, it will not survive. Yet, where have business people been taught innovation? They have had to learn it on their own in order to survive the economic pressures of a competitive society.

"We believe that innovation and creativity can be

developed in anyone. The old belief was that only a few individuals were highly gifted with creativity, and the average person just had to get along without it. This is totally incorrect, and an example of switched-off thinking. Unfortunately, most children have their creativity punished out of them by a very young age. What is left by the time they get to school is quickly destroyed."

"What can our audience members do to access their creativity?"

"It helps to think of ourselves as having a creative muscle that must be exercised — otherwise it will atrophy. There are many ways to exercise our creative muscle. For example, we teach relaxation and visualization techniques to help the children quiet their minds and open up their imaginations. It is also very important to release judgment because it stops the creative flow immediately.

"There is a beautiful old story of a successful merchant who visited a great teacher to gain knowledge and understanding. The teacher offered him a cup of tea and continued pouring tea into the already full cup. 'Stop! Stop!' cried the man. The teacher replied, 'You are like this cup. You came here seeking understanding, but your mind is overflowing with all your own knowledge, beliefs, and prejudices. Before you can receive understanding, you must allow your mind to become empty.'"

"Steve, tell us more about emptying the mind."

"It's done by quieting the mind, letting go of presuppositions and judgments. Then we can see the world with a new set of eyes and listen with a new set of ears. For example, I used to have this notion that I wasn't a creative person. I thought the creative person in my life was my wife, and she encouraged that by kidding me about my clumsy attempts at being creative. Then one day I realized that I had plenty of creative ideas available to me, just as she did."

"Please explain."

"I started researching the subject and doing the brain/mind exercises we now use in Whole School. In addition, I began using my nondominant, or 'other' hand for writing and for things such as eating, shaving, combing my hair. What an interesting and enlightening experience!

"First of all, I would like to ask everyone to do what I did by writing your full name with your nondominant hand....

"As soon as you have finished, write with your dominant hand what you think of that signature."

"Do we have some feedback from our audience?"

Audience Member #2: "My right hand wrote the word 'juvenile.'"

Audience Member #3: "Mine was 'sloppy.'"

Audience Member #4: "And mine was 'stupid-looking.'"

"Please register your response at your console. How many of you wrote something negative or judgmental about the writing of your nondominant hand? Thank you for your participation. Our studio monitor shows that the responses of 89 percent of our audience were judgmental about their other hand. Do we have feedback from some of you who are in the 11 percent?"

Audience Member #5: "Well, I'm ambidextrous, so I can easily switch from one hand to the other."

Audience Member #6: "My response was that it looked childlike, but I didn't see that as negative."

Steve: "I love it! You're exactly right. Our other hand appears childlike because it's untrained and very new at writing, just like a child. The fascinating thing is that using our other hand is a way to open up little-used areas of our brain. For example, because each hemisphere of the brain controls the opposite side of the body, a right-handed person will normally be using the left brain a great deal of the time. When that same person begins to use the left hand, they access their right brain, which is considered to be the more creative side of the brain. And the childlike quality is the key! Children have a beginner's mind — they are always seeing the world with a new set of eyes because they are open to the wonder surrounding them. And they allow that childlike, playful self to find the magic in every experience. Just ask a three-year-old to describe the butterfly nearby or the grasshopper at her feet. We need to reawaken our sense of wonder in order to access who we really are! Uh ... I get kind of carried away on this subject."

"You communicate how important this is to you, Steve. Tell us more about your experience with using your nondominant hand."

"Well, my commitment was to use my other hand for everything possible for three months. Imagine maneuvering chopsticks with your left hand to eat noodles and stir fry! It does take practice. What started happening was truly a reawakening for me. As time passed, my creative skills returned. Drawing was easier with my left hand than with my right. I also began to experience ideas flowing into my awareness that were good, workable, and innovative. Basically what the other-hand experience did for me was to teach me to trust my intuition and believe that I could be as creative as I would allow myself to be. By using my other hand, I bypassed judgment and prejudice and allowed my creative muscle to begin working again."

"Do your students enjoy this exercise?"

"They love it! It is a way to keep them exercising their creative muscle. Most importantly, I need to emphasize that their creative projects are never, never criticized, or judged by any 'normal' standards for their grade level. They are allowed free reign of their imagination, and as a result, they are trusting themselves on a deeper, more intuitive level. When that happens, they trust others more implicitly. And when children grow up trusting themselves and others, they are more responsible, self-actualized citizens."

"Did you want to mention any other experiences that encourage creativity?"

"Yes. Mind mapping is a wonderful tool to help us think more creatively. The process involves writing the main idea we want to develop in the center of a page and drawing a circle around this idea. Place different ideas that relate to the main thought on branches or arms extending from the circle. Develop each idea with supporting information, also extending from the main branches. It is very helpful to use a different color for each main branch. Mind mapping by-passes the linear, left-brain thinking and opens up right-brain processes. Withhold judgment of any ideas until the mind map is complete. Then use the map to create your project.

"Mind mapping can also be used for note taking, and there is usually an 80 percent better retention than with the traditional outline method of note taking. Again, be sure to use different colors for each group of ideas that branch from the main topic."

"Thank you, Steve, for your excellent ideas on the creative process. I wish you continued success as you develop your Whole School program. We have more questions from the audience."

Audience Member #7: "I'm a fifth grade teacher, and I can't believe your airy-fairy, permissive attitude toward kids. We've got to show them who's boss, or we'll raise a nation of juvenile delinquents!"

Steve: "My question for you is, 'Who is the boss?' In the business world, the customer is always the boss. Why don't we think of the children and their parents as the customers and build a partnership relationship with them instead of running our classes by intimidation and dominance?"

Audience Member #7: "I don't care how you describe

your Utopia — we still have to teach discipline."

Steve: "What were you told about discipline problems as a new teacher?"

Audience Member #7: "I remember being told to expect problems."

Steve: "We always find what we're looking for because the world is our mirror. In Whole School, we aren't looking for discipline problems, so we don't cause them by our negative expectations.

"We never use the word 'discipline.' It's interesting that this word keeps coming up when we're talking about learning and creativity. Discipline is derived from the word 'disciple.' The dictionary defines disciple as 'a person who subscribes to the teachings of a master and assists in spreading them.' When you take the creative minds of children and force them to subscribe to the teachings of a master — an underpaid and often undermotivated teacher — you are murdering creativity and fostering robots. We welcome children who do not fit the norm.

"If we do have a child who gets into frequent conflict, we counsel with them and their parents about their diet and their emotional environment. An unhealthy diet will often cause hyperactivity or depression, as will an unhealthy emotional environment. If they are eating junk food with food dyes and chemical additives, we recommend a healthier alternative. We teach nutrition in our classes and in our lunchroom, where we serve wholesome, balanced meals that are chemical-free. We also have bottled drinking water so that the children aren't drinking chemically-treated water."

Audience Member #8: "But you can't possibly believe that kids aren't going to behave violently. I mean, they learn these behaviors by watching television, and you can't as a teacher control that, can you?"

Steve: "When we interview prospective candidates and their parents, we have a strict requirement that parents monitor what their children watch on television. The selective viewing process keeps them from being programmed by what we call 'junk food for the mind.' Another vital part of our agreement with parents and students is that our students will not play war games either on our playground or at home. We want our children to learn to solve conflict peacefully, but if they grow up playing with guns, then they learn to prepare for war. I recently saw a toddler who was holding a toy pistol. His mother was praising him every time he pulled the trigger. When we give children war toys, we are teaching a war mentality."

Audience Member #8: "But aren't you living in a totally unrealistic world? If kids are kept in this positive cocoon until they get out of school, how will they ever handle the real world?"

Steve: "This concept of learning, as it spreads, will empower the children to change their world so that it becomes a mirror for their holistic thinking."

Audience Member #9: "Are your students screened for intelligence?"

Steve: "No, we take all levels, including children that have been called 'learning disabled,' provided they are willing, with their parents, to take responsibility for the partnership of learning. There are no learning disabled children, only learning disabled teaching methods. We believe that all kids in our program have an equal chance of succeeding, regardless of their I.Q."

Audience Member #9: "Are you saying that some kids aren't smarter than others?"

Steve: "Children learn in different ways and in different environments. Einstein was at one time considered to be mentally retarded. We provide the optimum learning environment for each child."

Audience Member #8: "Yeah, what about Einstein? All your creativity tricks don't begin to compare to the great scientific knowledge that Einstein and others are responsible for."

Steve: "I'm so glad you asked that question! Do you know how he developed the theory of relativity? He spent two hours imagining that he was riding a lightning bolt through the universe, and the result was his famous formula, $E=mc^2$. He stated that imagination was more important than knowledge and also that his understanding of the universe did not come from his rational mind. He is the perfect example of a person who was able to translate his creativity into action. That is what we are accomplishing in Whole School."

Audience Member #10: "Aren't you talking about a Utopian dream?"

Steve: "Dreams give birth to reality, and Utopia is working, as long as we use our *Owner's Manuals* and honor the amazing potential in each individual. There is a very creative person inside each of us. As we use our wholebrain, we access our creativity by accepting it and using it to improve the quality of our lives."

"Thank you, Steve, for your participation, and thank you, Rhonda and Helen. Your leadership and example are the pathways of the future. Thank you to our audience for joining us today in Uniqueland.

"It is time to become better acquainted with your own creativity. Think of a question that is concerning you about your personal life, your relationships, or your job.... Now close your eyes and take some deep breaths, releasing any tension that you are holding in your body.

"Allow your mind to take you to the shore of a beautiful lake. There is a small boat waiting for you, and you get in, seating yourself comfortably. Mysteriously, the boat begins to move toward an unknown destination, and you relax in the understanding that you are totally safe. Feel the gentle breeze caressing your hair, your cheeks. Listen to the sounds of the waves lapping

against the side of the boat.

"*Soon you notice that it is getting darker and that you are moving slowly through an underground waterway. Sense the warm darkness enveloping you in its comforting embrace. There is light appearing at the end of the passage — bright sunshine. As the boat moves into this light, you see a beautiful cove ahead of you and the figures of two people standing on the shore. Drawing closer, you observe that one of them is a young child — a child that looks very much like you. Now the boat is waiting at the shore while you step easily onto dry land. The little child takes your hand, and together you go on a voyage of discovery, stopping to examine rocks and butterflies, tiny fish near the shore, and the lush vegetation — all through the delighted eyes of the young child....*

"*Hand in hand, you and the child approach the figure waiting by the boat. Together you ask the question that you have been pondering. This wise entity very lovingly responds to your question and then assists you and the child into the boat. Cradling the child in your arms, you begin your return, confident in the understanding that you have been given an answer that you will remember at the right moment.*

"*The return is rapid, and you invite the child to remain at your side to help you see the world through the eyes of wonderment. When you are ready, return to the present space and time....*

"*Within each of us there is a magical, childlike, creative self who is waiting to be welcomed back into our lives. We can choose to honor this creative self, making our lives an expression of our uniqueness.*

"*This is Maya Cristal, inviting you to join us next week for 'High Performance Adventure,' when our subject will be the 'Conscious Living Adventure.' Our guests are Micheline Holiday, founder of the Center for Conscious Living in the Colorado Rocky Mountains, and a panel of ten-year-old children who will answer questions on their involvement in making peace with the Planet Earth. What will it mean to you to gain tools to help you live more consciously in partnership with the Earth? It is a matter of assuring that we have a sustainable future.*

"Until then, remember to nurture your creative self, and you will unleash a powerful force in your life. Your future and that of this planet depend on your choosing to access your creativity."

Announcer: "You may obtain a written transcript of this program and a corresponding Creativity Brainware package by calling the number appearing on your television screen."

Chapter 23

A Step Backwards Into the Future

Maya responded to her harmonic frequency with a knowing smile. She had pre-programmed her Dreamtime to take her forward in space and time to the latter part of the 21st Century. She experienced no surprise when the image of a young child appeared before her, sleeping on a soft, billowy cloud. Maya noticed the innocence and wisdom in the startling green eyes that fluttered open. "You are the one called Maya."

"Yes, I am."

"Your mission is my destiny." Maya watched in awe as the child's image was transforming, first into an older child, gradually into a young adult, and finally into an ancient woman whose face was stained with tears. Then in an instant, the face was again that of a child.

"You may recognize me by other names, but please call me Gaia. I am the embodiment of the life cycle of the Living Spaceship Earth. What you have witnessed gives you an image of the changes that are now occurring. The Planet Earth has been undergoing a rapid transformation similar to a rebirthing process. The sorrow in the ancient face was caused by various factors, primarily exploitation by humankind. Now that awareness is returning, the planet is being reborn. Would you like to have a glimpse into the future?"

Maya nodded in silent agreement.

"All is in readiness," replied Gaia. "Come with me."

A shaft of brilliant light pierced the darkening sky surrounding Maya and her guide. Suddenly a path appeared — a glowing ribbon of light across the universe. Maya followed Gaia, walking across a field of stars, shimmering like diamond dust. Their light-path took them through a whirlwind, sweeping them up into a shower of fiery lights, illuminating the inky blackness of a moonless sky. And then, she heard Gaia's gentle voice, "Maya, I will leave you. With your next awareness, you will know that the future is now."

Δ Δ Δ

Maya gazed around her in joyous disbelief. This looks like a paradise, like Mayata, but I know it is the Living Spaceship Earth. She was standing in the middle of a lush, garden setting. Natural grasses and wildflowers formed a thick carpet of brilliant color, surrounded by a myriad of trees, many bearing fruit. There was a blur of movement through the dense foliage. She stepped forward to get a closer look and caught glimpses of vehicles moving silently along what appeared to be an electronic roadway. She looked up at the clear blue sky in amazement. There are no signs of air pollution, and this place is like a wilderness area, but it is apparently in the middle of a city. I must talk to some Earthlings to discover what has occurred.

Approaching her were two runners, a woman and a man. Maya smiled a greeting, but they were too engrossed in their thought transference to notice her. She began running beside them, telepathically requesting information. The woman's eyes widened in amazement. Then she nodded in agreement, discussing the memory access mode with her partner.

"There is a presence of advanced harmonic frequency who would like to join us, Tom."

"Yes, of course," he smiled.

"Everything appears transformed. What has happened to the Living Spaceship Earth?" Maya asked eagerly.

"Many changes have occurred since our grandparents, and even our parents experienced a time of major upheaval on this planet," the woman who introduced herself as Sterling replied. "On the one hand, peace was breaking out everywhere, and on the other hand, frightened individuals were clinging to old habit patterns, almost immobilized by the massive transformation surrounding them. Many people reacted with fear and denial."

"Yeah," added Tom. "Things had to change. The air was so polluted that some of the larger cities had major health problems caused by ecodiseases. The outcome of continuous air alerts was a mobilization of the former military forces to clean up the environment. 'Individual response-ability for a sustainable future' was the motto of the day. My grandparents volunteered to serve in a grassroots movement called the Gaia Project and were involved in the reclaiming of natural wilderness areas such as this one."

"What was done about the problem of starvation?"

Sterling replied, "Once people got involved in cleaning up the planet, they opened their awareness to the hunger crisis. The Gaia Project expanded to teach responsibility for family planning and radical evolution of food consumption styles. We in the U.S. have learned that a mostly vegetarian diet is much healthier for ourselves and for the planet. No longer are rainforests burned to provide grazing land for cattle so we can eat hamburgers and steaks. It just doesn't make sense to be destroying our natural resources for the sake of a self-centered, unhealthy lifestyle."

"Don't forget the birth control issue," added Tom. "Certain religious groups used to tell their followers that it was their duty to have as many children as possible. That contributed greatly to overpopulation and starvation. Our generation finds it hard to believe that a couple would obey a religion that dictated that they could not practice birth control. Of course, that was all part of the patriarchal religious exploitation of women that went on for centuries. Now men consider themselves partners with women, and it's beautiful!" He touched Sterling's hand lovingly. "We realize that feminine energy is nurturing and intuitive, and we honor that side of both women and men. As a man, I can choose to be nurturing rather than aggressive. I'm aware of the need for balance between the masculine and feminine energy in each of us."

Sterling added, "Because of the spirit of cooperation that came about just in time to save our Earth home, we have found ways to live in harmony with each other and with the planet. Peace is a way of life, as opposed to the wars and aggression of the past. Since there is no need to spend billions of dollars on national defense, the environment and education are now top priorities for government spending."

A group of school children came into view, laughing and playing in the center of the wooded area. "Is it a holiday?" Maya asked.

"No," Sterling replied. "Children spend one day a week on nature studies, learning to respect and conserve the Earth's resources. Being in harmony with nature is very important to us."

"That's true," Tom added. "We never want things to deteriorate as they did in the past. I believe we've learned our lesson!"

"What caused the changes?"

Sterling answered, "People started opening their eyes and using their brains in a balanced way. They became aware of their *Owner's Manuals* and started making responsible choices. No longer was technology looked upon as the answer to all problems. Our grandparents were part of the generation that opened their minds to the path of the heart. The result was the awakening and empowerment of individuals who realized that they had to make a difference and create a better life for themselves and future generations."

"I do not see smokestacks or autos with exhaust fumes. What form of energy is being used to fuel industry and transportation?"

Sterling responded, "An advanced form of electricity which utilizes the energy of the sun, the wind, ocean currents, and most recently, an energy derived from molecular conversion without the danger of the old fashioned nuclear power. We're still having to safeguard nuclear waste from the late 20th Century. That's a problem that every generation must contend with. It's unbelievable that nuclear power was not banned worldwide until almost the end of the last century."

"What happened in the 'third world countries?'"

"That term has not been used for years," replied Tom. "I suppose you could say that there are only first world countries. It only took about fifty years to bring about world equality once the threat of war was eliminated."

"What happened to autocratic forms of government?"

"It was as though everything changed overnight," Sterling replied. "Dictators could not rule without fear and intimidation. When fear was released by acceptance of personal responsibility, the dictators were ousted by popular demand."

"What challenges does your society face today?"

"We're still advancing technologically. The worldwide language has helped to eliminate most misunderstandings," continued Sterling. "There is still the challenge of interpreting inter-Galactic transmissions, but there is no danger in communications with advanced beings from other systems. Societies that send space travelers are beyond violence."

"What about religions?"

"Again, the word 'religion' is rarely used except in a historical context," explained Sterling. "When people rediscovered their own personal power and self-worth, they lost their need to be dominated by any outside authority figures. There was very little bitterness involved as people began to embrace a more tolerant spirituality. Many of the religious buildings are now used as spiritual centers."

"What would you describe as the most important problem facing humankind?"

"I can answer that," laughed Tom. "Probably boredom. The many technological advances in areas such as robotics have made life too easy. It's high entertainment for us to watch the old videos of the late 20th and early 21st Centuries. But when it gets to looking like those were 'the good old days,' we remember all the problems that were a part of that time — like disease."

"What is the disease situation now?"

"There is no disease," continued Tom. "It was gradually given up, as people have taken responsibility for their own wellness. All that remains of the old medical paradigm is maintenance and repair of our human bodies."

"What is the average life expectancy, Tom?"

"Approximately one hundred years. Transition is normally a conscious choice. Some choose to live to 130 or 140, but only when they are highly motivated by a special project. Most are anxious to time-space travel to other galaxies and ..."

"Tom, you appear puzzled," Sterling stated. "Is something wrong?"

"No, something is terribly right! I've just experienced a flashback. Maya, you seem very familiar to me — like we've met before. My memory is of a myriad of feelings and voices — no pictures. It had something to do with bicycles and intuition — and then the most peaceful calm imaginable."

Maya squeezed Tom's hand and smiled across forever. "You will remember fully when the time is right for you. You are special, Tom."

Hugging them both, Maya said, "Thank you for sharing your world with me." She knew she had experienced tomorrow — a tomorrow that she must assure.

Δ Δ Δ

As Maya slipped gently away on her five harmonic tones, she saw once again the sad eyes of Gaia as an ancient woman, the embodiment of the Living Spaceship Earth, suffering great agony. Maya spoke with love and compassion, "It will not be long now, Gaia. You will smile soon."

Chapter 24

The Conscious Living Adventure

"**G**ood Evening. This is Maya Cristal, your host for 'High Performance Adventure.' Our program this evening is the 'Conscious Living Adventure.' Tonight's Brainware will provide you with tools to live in balance and harmony with the Planet Earth. You will enjoy our panel of ten-year-old children who will discuss their active involvement in the return to ecobalance.

"Our first guest is the chairperson of the President's Council for a Sustainable Environment. She is also involved in numerous non-profit organizations that are taking action to balance the Earth's fragile ecology. She is the founder of the Center for Conscious Living in the Colorado Rocky Mountains and a recent space traveler. Please welcome Micheline Holiday."

"Hello, Maya. Thank you for inviting me to be on your show. You are touching many lives and raising the consciousness on this planet."

"Thank you, Micheline. I have been looking forward to your appearance on our program because of your leadership in environmental action. What influenced you to found the Center for Conscious Living?"

"My life has been a series of events that have led me to this project. I grew up in Belgium, where my father was a musician, and my mother ran the family import-export business. Both of them were on the road much of the time because of business and also because of their stormy relationship. Being an only child, I was pulled between the two of them, and spent my time traveling with first one, and then the other. Both had an intense passion for life, which they passed on to me. My father also taught me a deep love and respect for nature.

"I came to the United States to attend Southern Cal during the 1980's. You can imagine the education I received! When my mother became aware of the liberal environment I was in, she immediately sent for me to come home. Instead, I married my sweetheart and moved to Southern Colorado with him to farm. We raised cattle and raised children. It was a good life, rich with love and opportunities to grow together. Then our youngest daughter became very ill. The doctors diagnosed her as having leukemia, but we refused to accept that as a terminal sentence.

"Because of her illness, I started reading everything I could find concerning nutrition and the role of the mind in healing. It was a gradual awakening process for us. Susie lived four years longer than the doctors had predicted. She taught us many lessons on the value of each precious moment, and she taught us the true meaning of unconditional love. Because of our new awareness of the role of diet in health, we decided to sell our cattle and began the process of conversion to organic farming. We realized that the hormone-filled feed we had been using for our cattle was carcinogenic, as were the pesticides we had been using on our crops. We also became aware that these chemicals represented a system of dominance of the Earth and her creatures by humankind — a system we could no longer support."

"That must have been a dramatic awakening — one that transformed your lives."

"Yes, it did. Bill and I worked night and day to organize a non-profit organization that would help raise the awareness level in our country and throughout the world. We wanted to reverse the tide of thousands of years of human aggression against the Earth.

"Then one icy January night, we were involved in a terrible accident. I was driving on a winding, mountain road and suddenly lost control of our pickup. We went over the edge of the mountain and rolled our truck seven times before stopping upside down in a dry creek bed. I broke my back and my left leg, and Bill, well ... he never regained consciousness. He died three days later."

"I feel your sadness and pain. How have you dealt with this loss?"

"At first I felt only guilt and bitterness. I blamed myself, and then I started wondering how he could leave me just when things were starting to pull together with the farm and with our Gaia Project plans. Then a friend recommended that wellness counseling would help release those feelings."

"What about your own injury?"

"Well, I had back surgery, and when the doctors told me that I would never walk again, I told them they were crazy! They fused my spine and put a pin in my leg. That was just over four years ago, and I'm just as physically active now, if not more so than before the accident. I ski, ride my mountain bicycle, and swim. The doctors said I was the closest thing to a paraplegic they had ever seen."

"You are a courageous woman, Micheline."

"Thank you, Maya. I consider myself more persevering than courageous. I have a dream to fulfill."

"What is your dream?"

"I see humankind in a time of revolutionary change, a time for honoring all life forms, for a return to balance in our relationship with the planet. We're emerging from the aggressive stance of the past — the attitude that the Earth was here to serve our needs and that we could rape and plunder her resources as much as we wished. The change in attitude is a return to the ecological wisdom of ancient tribes who lived in harmony with nature. If we are to survive, and I believe that we will, we must accept the role of nurturers of our Earth home."

"I share that same dream, Micheline. Where do we begin?"

"All change begins with me, with you, with each individual. As we accept ourselves and live in partnership with the feminine and masculine energy within us, then and then only, can we live peacefully and in harmony with the Earth. But this change is not something we can sit around and just meditate about while we leave the job of active ecology to someone else. We must make a radical difference and do it now!"

"I can sense the urgency in what you are saying. What is the purpose of the Center for Conscious Living?"

"The purpose of our Center is to heighten awareness. We offer a place where concerned citizens from all over the world can come to attend forums and training programs on everything from self-actualization to conflict resolution and planetary consciousness. We have built a global community by donating portions of the 200,000 acre ranch to spiritual groups who live at the Center. They represent diverse backgrounds — from Carmelite Catholics to Zen and Tibetan Buddhist monks. In addition, a number of Native American tribes make pilgrimages to the land, which they say has been sacred for thousands of years. We have chapels, temples, sweat lodges, community buildings, organic and experimental gardens, streams, mountains, and more deer than people. The land is a complete ecosystem. It's a virtual wilderness in its pure state with underground rivers, hot springs, and there's still gold in the mountains."

"What projects are ongoing at the Center?"

"A major project has been to use sustainable energy sources. For example, our heat comes from geothermal energy from our underground hot springs, and we also convert our garbage into power through the process of biomass.

"We have a solar farming community, another project that is developing a sustainable, high-altitude agricultural system, a holistic health center, a hermitage, and the Spiritual Life Institute. We are constantly looking for groups and individuals who want to discover alternate choices for a healthy planet."

"Who is 'we?'"

"My two sons have worked with me to develop the Center from the original Gaia Project days."

"Micheline, I applaud your active involvement in the return to ecobalance. You recently returned from a space expedition. Tell us about your experiences."

"This was the most exciting adventure of my life! I had always dreamed of participating in a space expedition. The opportunity was the result of my contact with several NASA scientists who visited the Center. They were concerned that we handle our space exploration in an environmentally sensitive way. They invited me to apply for an intensive training program in Houston, and I was chosen to participate in the most recent mission."

"What was your most memorable adventure in space?"

"I'm glad you asked, because somehow — I can't explain it, but I feel it had something to do with you. One day while I was at the permanent space station, I saw a bright light moving very slowly, and I watched as it came in my general direction. Then I had a vision of being on a different planet. I distinctly remember seeing two moons in the sky. I was walking in the direction of the light, and wandered into a deserted city, surrounded by a garden of huge crystals. I sat down to rest for a minute and began to sense the brightness surrounding me. I felt no fear, only curiosity. Then it was as though ... it's hard to put into words."

"Take your time."

"Well, in this dream or vision or whatever it was, I was face to face with a tall being with flowing blond hair, dressed in a white tunic, with a coral snake wrapped around each wrist. He gave me a message that he said I was supposed to deliver, but I have no idea what it meant or who the message was for."

"What was the message?"

"He said, 'Tell her to take the path through the fire.' When I tried to ask him what he meant, he disappeared in a cloud of rainbow-colored lights.... Maya, are you all right?"

"Yes ... yes, was there something else?"

"No, that was all I could remember when I came back to reality, except for one more thing."

"Yes?"

"I have never experienced such unconditional love as I did in that moment."

"Thank you ... Micheline ... thank you....

"We have questions from our audience, but first I have a question for each of you to answer at your consoles. Are you taking personal action to return the Planet Earth to ecobalance? Thank you for your responses. My monitor shows a 93 percent 'Yes' response.

"Please give us some feedback."

Audience Member #1: "I'm not really worried about all this global stuff. It just sounds like a lot of media hype to me, and besides, what difference does it make what one person does?"

Micheline: "That's exactly the toxic thinking that has gotten us into such ecological imbalance. Change has to start with each individual making a difference!"

Audience Member #2: "I think you're being entirely too optimistic about the future. At the rate the rainforests are disappearing, and the acid rain and all the other poisons are destroying our air, we on Planet Earth only have a few years before life as we know it is going to be destroyed. I've already built an underground shelter to try to save my family and myself."

Micheline: "I agree that we must operate from a sense of extreme urgency, and yet I feel that we need to come from a place of love rather than a place of fear. As we put aside our nationalism and work together with other countries in a spirit of cooperation, we will be able to bring about a peace and a healing of the Earth."

Audience Member #3: "I heard you say something about a global community and world peace. The more peace breaks out, the more military we put out of a job!"

Micheline: "The dictionary defines military as 'of or pertaining to war.' Do we really want to support a war mentality? Why don't we rename the military and armed forces organizations and put them to work on peaceful missions — cleaning up the planet? Why is it important to have an enemy? The only thing we have to fear — our only enemy — is fear. Is it too simple an answer to replace fear with love? War with peace? Ecodisaster with ecobalance?"

Audience Member #4: "Your suggestion is preposterous! As an officer in the United States Navy, and a member of an organization called The Human Economics Movement, I'm concerned with what I see on TV and read in the newspapers. I told my wife just the other day, 'The good Lord created this planet, gave it to us to rule and subdue, and it's up to us to refashion it so that humans do not lose their position of superiority!'"

Micheline: "I beg you to wake up before it's too late! There are two attitudes that are killing us. One is apathy — the attitude that says, 'It's not my problem!' and the other is your attitude of aggression. It is because of all the years of humankind's, or should I use the more accurate term, 'mankind's,' refashioning the world to meet human needs that we are in such trouble. We need to release the idea of superiority of humans over all other living beings. That is old paradigm, toxic thinking! We need to accept that we are one with all of nature and return to balance and harmony with the Earth."

Audience Member #4: "That's bullshit, lady! I want to warn you, Dr. Maya Cristal. We're fed up with all this environment-first nonsense. We're tired of your doomsayer environmentalism. All you have done is cause trouble for human economics! We've had enough of your *Owner's Manual,* too!"

Audience Member #5: "Nonsense! I agree with what Micheline is saying. As a minister of a Christian Church, I was taught to believe that humans are superior to all other life forms, but that concept has been very damaging to our Earth home. There is a movement in religious organizations toward ecotheology, aligning our theology with the concern for a sustainable future. My church has been active for years in recycling and in offering educational seminars on planetary consciousness."

Audience Member #6: "I'm embarrassed by all the verbal rhetoric I've been hearing today. All I've heard is talk, talk, talk! What can I do *now* to make a difference? I believe in what you are saying, but give us something concrete to do, not just superficial platitudes!"

Micheline: "Thank you for your impassioned plea. I agree that we need action steps, yet conscious living must begin with an attitude change. For example, before purchasing anything, we need to make a conscious choice by asking some questions. How was the product manufactured? Were animals used for testing in the research and development of this product? Does the company conform to environmental standards? How is the product packaged? Can the product be recycled, or will it make more waste for our burgeoning landfills?

"If it's a food product, where was it produced? Did it have to be shipped — meaning a truck brought it a long distance. Is the product available from local food growers? Can it be purchased in bulk, so that there is less packaging waste?

"Don't support companies that are environmentally unconscious, but tell the management why you are not buying that product. Ask them to stop stocking it. When enough people make the same request, store managers will listen."

Audience Member #7: "You've got to be kidding! Before I buy a package of razor blades, I've got to go to the trouble to think through all those questions? I'd never get home from the store!"

Micheline: "Once this thought process becomes a habit, it only takes a few seconds. If we don't go to the trouble to think about it — and take action — we are living unconsciously. By the way, please purchase a reusable razor instead of the disposable ones.

"Each of you will receive an Ecological Action Guide as part of today's Brainware, with detailed instructions on how to do your part in bringing our beautiful Living Spaceship Earth back to her deserved balance. Many of you are already following these action steps, but I will recap a few of them.

"Recycle every possible resource: bottles, cans, plastics, paper products of all forms — not just newspapers — batteries, automobile oil, car parts. Compost food scraps, ashes, grass clippings, leaves, animal waste. Eliminate toxic household cleansers by purchasing environmentally-friendly products. Take toxic materials to special recycling centers to be disposed of — do not throw toxic materials such as batteries in the trash to be taken to landfills. They end up seeping toxins into our ground water supplies.

"Precycle by purchasing products that are not heavily packaged. Do not purchase products packaged in styrofoam or plastic. Buy food in bulk. Reuse paper bags. Better yet, buy several cloth or string shopping bags, and take them with you every time you shop. Europeans have been doing this for years.

"Carry a guide with you whenever you shop that identifies products that are environmentally safe and that don't use animal testing. Such guides are available at your bookstore. Purchase products that are labeled 'green' because you will be supporting companies that are taking responsible action for the environment.

"Conserve resources like water, food, soap, gasoline, air conditioning, heat, and electricity. Every home should have a cistern to catch the rain and snow runoff for future lawn watering, car washing, and washing machines. Autos that get less than one hundred miles per gallon will soon be taxed heavily. Free, or at least low-cost transportation is a must for cities. Even cross country travel should be done in multi-units. It sounds so basic, but carpool or ride a bicycle whenever possible.

"Refuse to accept junk mail or junk fax mail. Request the removal of your name from mailing lists. I used to get hundreds of junk pieces every month before I put a stop to this ridiculous waste by returning the mail or calling each company's toll free number.

"One of the greatest advances recently has been the closing of nuclear power sites. As these sites are totally shut down, our next challenge is to safely locate and store the nuclear wastes that were dumped for so many years. Of course, other energy sources, like fossil fuels, are being rapidly eliminated due to incentives offered by most countries.

"Now for the items requiring the true changing of habits. Our eating habits must be altered. Little or no meat consumption would do more to bring balance to our environment than any other single change. People live longer and healthier on a diet of whole grains, nuts, fruits, and vegetables. The conversion of grains to animal protein is no longer justifiable with the exception of fish and fowl, which most of us believe will always retain its acceptable food chain status.

"Certain things must stop, like fast food restaurants using disposable cups, containers, and eating utensils. The quickest way to accomplish this is to boycott environmentally irresponsible establishments. The world's largest hamburger chain has shown a loss for the past three years due to its continued involvement in the purchase of foreign beef, raised on land that used to be tropical rainforests. I repeat, boycott these places! Do not support the destruction of the environment. The fastest growing, fast food restaurant chain has mostly vegetarian offerings that contain more protein and less cholesterol than any greasy hamburger!

"There are many excellent books on this subject. Consciousness is growing rapidly. One area that still is controversial is population growth. Within the next ten years, I predict that world population will start a gradual, then a more marked decline, due to the move by the International Conference of World Religions to have birth control accepted by all religious groups.

"Thanks again for your question. We must each choose to exercise our personal power by taking action to return the Earth to balance and harmony."

"Thank you, Micheline, for your beautiful example of conscious living.

"Next we have a group of guests who are excited to

join us. Please welcome our international panel of ten-year-olds: Margaret from Australia; Reshma from India; Nicholas from Russia; Jennifer from Chicago; and Robert, a Native American from New Mexico.

"I want to ask our panel the same questions we asked our audience. Are you taking personal action to return the Planet Earth to ecobalance? Please answer 'Yes' or 'No' at your consoles. My monitor shows a 100 percent 'Yes' response. Who will tell us why you said 'Yes?'"

Reshma: "It is a duty and an honor to be able to serve the Earth when she needs us. I want to learn how to make a better life for my people and make the Earth happy again."

Nicholas: "I was amazed at the apathy my parents told me about in the old days toward such serious issues. In my country, the adults were slow to wake up, also."

Jennifer: "Yeah, I hope everyone wakes up before it's too late. I want there to be a future."

"Thank you, panel. What can we do to conserve our natural resources?"

Margaret: "In my school in Melbourne we have been studying the effect of pollution on the ozone layer. Also, every Saturday, my brothers and I collect newspapers and take them to a recycling plant. My teacher told us that a pile of newspapers ten feet high will save one tree. Even though our city has curbside recycling, not everyone cares like we do. I'm also the editor for our school newspaper on the environment. It's called *Ecokids.*"

Jennifer: "I saw on TV that Americans used to dump tons and tons of disposable diapers in landfills each year. Wow! That's a lot of plastic that won't go away. My mom told me she began using a diaper service when I was born. She said it was really less expensive, and I'm proud of not being part of the problem."

Robert: "My grandfather taught me that we should

honor the Earth, but all I ever see is more and more highways and tourists invading our hills and leaving behind all their trash. One thing my grandfather has mentioned is that he has hope because many of the non-Native American people he has talked to lately are showing respect for the ways of native peoples. Some have even told him that they feel like they understand and respect my people's love for Mother Earth. It is sad that many of my people have forgotten the old ways."

Nicholas: "We need to understand each other and work together."

"How can we do this?"

Nicholas: "When I get older, I plan to come to the United States to live with an American family and go to school. Then I am going to be a teacher in my country."

Margaret: "Last year my family spent our vacation in Mexico City. We had lots of fun because we worked with a co-op group from many countries, planting trees and cleaning up trash. One of my Mexican friends wrote to me and said that we made a big difference there."

Audience Member #8: "These children are young and idealistic. What do they know about world problems?"

Reshma: "You may find us idealistic, but what are you doing to make a difference?"

Audience Member #8: "I make a decent living. I'm looking after my family, and I let the government look after its own problems."

Reshma: "It is too bad you feel that way. I *am* my government. Sometimes I do not look forward to growing up. Adults complicate simple matters so much."

"Thank you, panel. You have offered us some simple truths that are part of using our Owner's Manuals to make intelligent choices for a sustainable future. Do not let anyone prevent you from remaining actively involved in the return to ecobalance."

Maya moved among the panel members, hugging

each child in an embrace of love and appreciation.

"*Healing the planet must begin with inner healing for each individual. Please close your eyes, take some deep breaths, and allow your mind and body to relax. Now imagine that you are a traveler on a space mission. Buckle yourself into your seat, hear the roar of the engines, and feel the surge of power that lifts you off the ground. You adjust rapidly to the changing gravity and move to the window. In the distance you see a beautiful planet, blue-green in color, floating in a sea of sky. Visualize the Earth in her perfection, sparkling like a jewel in the dark blue cosmos.*

"*Imagine for a few moments that you are the Planet Earth, that you have undergone immense change, much of it traumatic, but that the pain is a part of the past. Experience the joy of knowing that your human inhabitants are reawakening, remembering their bond with you, and accepting that they are one with all life forms.*

"*Now travel on the wind over the oceans, much cleaner now than in the last century.... Visit a rainforest, knowing that your conscious action is protecting many species from extinction. Spend some time walking down a forest path, surrounded by a curtain of green, smelling the richness of moist earth after a tropical rainstorm....*

"*Return your awareness to your life. Plan the additional steps you will take to show your love and respect for the Planet Earth.... See yourself remembering that each individual action does make a difference. Know that the healing of the Planet Earth is a mirror of the healing you are personally experiencing through using your Owner's Manual.... When you are ready, bring your awareness back to the present space and time, and open your eyes.*

"*Thank you, Micheline and the members of our panel, Margaret, Reshma, Nicholas, Jennifer, and Robert. Thank you to our audience for joining us and for your participation.*

"Please join us next week for 'High Performance Adventure,' when our topic will be the 'Transformation Adventure.' Our guests are Dr. Leo Townsend, a consultant in the field of change management; Connie Philips, former president of a Midwest bank holding company; and healer, Sierra Moreno. Look forward to these guests who will assist you in dealing with change from a position of strength.

"This is Maya Cristal reminding you to make a difference on this planet. Be a part of the solution — not a part of the problem."

Announcer: "You may obtain a written transcript of this program and a corresponding Conscious Living Brainware package by calling the number appearing on your television screen."

Chapter 25

The Path Through the Fire

Maya got into the taxi, experiencing a vague uneasiness. She intuitively knew that this taxi ride was a dangerous choice, yet she was certain that she was following the path that would lead to her destiny. She had not mentioned to Rich, or anyone, the threatening phone call she had received minutes prior to the start of the program. Rich had become increasingly protective since the first death-threat letter several weeks ago. Now she had slipped out the side door of the station to avoid the crowd of fans and the usual ride home in the security car. She shunned the notoriety of being a superstar.

The angry voice on the phone had accused her of being a false messiah and a witch. "Such power as you advocate does not belong to humans," the caller had raged. "We want you to burn in hell!"

Maya remembered the words of a philosopher of the 20th Century who had stated, "We are all Gods in the chrysalis." Why are these people afraid of my message of power balanced with love? What do they have to lose

— their control over others? To live a life committed to fulfilling one's highest purpose cannot be considered evil, except by those who are ruled by fear.

The taxi driver did not glance up as Maya closed the door and gave him her address. He nodded and moved into the heavy traffic. The ride home after a program was a time for solitude and reflection on what had been accomplished. This time, there was no blaring radio, no attempt at mundane conversation by the driver, only silence, as the miles passed by.

Lost in reverie, Maya was jolted to reality as the driver passed her turnoff, taking instead the road that led to Thunder Mountain. "Where are you going? Please turn around now!"

The driver responded by ignoring her and pressing down on the accelerator, tires squealing as he raced around the curves. Moments later, he slammed on the brakes, screeching to a stop. The doors on either side of Maya opened, and two people, dressed in black, with masked faces, jumped in. Rather than struggling to escape, she centered her awareness. The next moment, she felt something needle-sharp and painful entering her arm, and she slumped over in the seat.

Δ Λ Δ

Maya lay on a cot in a tiny, cell-like room, floating through a maze of hallucinogenic states — shadowy memories, scattered images filling her senses. Light and darkness filtered through a prism of blue, green, rose, violet and gold, lifting her on its hues.

Starchild with a mission — a mission of power balanced with love. Running, running ever faster toward my friend and twin soul, Cyruse — together through time and space. In the jungle now, running beneath a ceiling of green. Keep the dream — much to be done. Mother and Father deeply concerned ... the fate of "perfect" beings. Carlos, coral snakes on his wrists, "Take the path through the fire ... path through the fire." My essence will live forever.

The sobs of Gaia — it will be soon, Gaia. You will smile again. A gentle face filled with concern and love, "How can you be so calm, Maya?"

I have chosen this test.... Through the fire — the path through the fire. "We want you to burn in hell" — "there are no barriers to those who release their fear." I am here for the return to balance and harmony of the Living Spaceship Earth. Mission *Owner's Manual* is raising awareness ... conscious living ... ecobalance.

Darkness, night — the Tree — one bird remaining, an enormous owl ... flying gently toward me, nestled in my arms. "You are the perfect balance of feminine and masculine energy — we call you Equadeity — Goddess and God, a partnership of balance and understanding. Merging wisdom — we are one. Transformation is now...."

Five harmonic tones, blended in absolute harmony — the gifts of Power, Love, Healing, Wisdom, and Understanding. A mirror of their perfection — they must remember their nobility. Getting closer now — the path ... the path through the fire. Snakes around my wrists, writhing, flowing into the flames ... rising higher and higher. My crystal self grows cloudy and dark, the object of hatred and fear. I have been here before. Warlords destroying life in the name of their God.

Truth can never be destroyed. Almost time ... the future is now ... Mission *Owner's Manual* is a transformational tool. It will not be long now, Gaia. You will smile soon. Healing is balance and harmony, our sacred right. The path opens before me — this is my choice — the path of the heart....

Δ Δ Δ

Maya returned to full consciousness with her head aching and her body strangely heavy. Slowly the memory of her taxi ride returned. Who were her masked captors, and what did they hope to accomplish? Were these the people who had been threatening her?

She felt a dull pain in her right shoulder. Then she remembered being half carried, half dragged from the taxi. One of her captors had crushed her shoulder against the wall as he opened a door. His companion, a woman whom he had called Roz, had gruffly ordered, "Be careful! We don't want to damage the prisoner before we get her confession on tape."

Maya took herself to alpha awareness to perform a healing visualization. First she saw a cleansing light entering her body at her spine, purifying every cell of the toxic drug she had been given. Then she concentrated on the muscular region of her bruised shoulder, feeling the warm, healing energy relax the soreness. She completed the process by balancing her energy centers.

Getting up from the cot, she performed some brain integration movements and full-body stretches. Totally centered and prepared for the unknown, she walked toward the door of the cell. Just as she reached to open it, the door burst open, and Maya stood facing her astonished captor, who said, "She's awake! Hurry, Roz!"

"What's wrong, Paul?" A woman's voice questioned from outside the cell.

"Is it time yet, Roz?"

"How many times do I have to tell you — not until she's made the tape and until I've played with her brain on the Jammer." The woman, Roz, appeared behind Paul, pointing an Uzi machine gun at Maya. "Just in case you try to get clever, Sweetie. Now, follow me."

Paul grabbed Maya's arm and pushed her down a long hallway into a brightly lit room, equipped with computers, a large control panel, and other equipment that she recognized as electronic brain experimentation devices. The equipment had been banned from use because the combination of electric shock and varying sound frequencies produced advanced hallucinogenic states, from which some of the early users had received permanent brain damage. She remembered reading of a scientist, Dr. Rosalyn Reichardt, who had used the equipment called the Brain Jammer to decode the subject's brain patterns, giving her total control over the repatterning which followed.

Maya looked into the steel gray eyes of Dr. Reichardt. "So, we meet at last, Princess Maya. That's what you are, aren't you, a princess from some far-away kingdom?"

Maya stared boldly into her cold eyes without responding.

"Come on, can't you defend yourself?"

"Truth needs no defense," Maya stated fearlessly.

"We'll see how well your truth protects you, Princess. Come, sit on your royal throne."

Maya was pushed and shoved roughly into the chair that dominated the room from its raised platform. Paul strapped her arms and legs so tightly that she had to focus on her breathing in order to keep from crying out from the pain. Then he pulled a rubber cap over her thick, long hair, placing a helmet-like headset over it, and attaching electrodes at her temples and at the base of her skull. "Welcome to your personal 'High Performance Adventure,'" mocked Roz.

Δ Δ Δ

Galactic Agent Josh waited impatiently outside Rich's office while the network owner and Rich carried on a heated discussion in the inner office.

"How could you let her leave on her own, Rich? For God's sake, this woman's our gold mine!"

"And how can you be so cold and unfeeling while Maya is in danger? Is money all you ever consider?" Rich shouted.

On the table lay a note that stated, "We have your 'High Performance Adventure' host. Cancel the program immediately. Make a nationally televised statement discrediting Maya Cristal by 10:00 p.m. tomorrow, or she will be killed. Do not call the Feds." The note was signed, "The Human Economics Movement."

"All right, all right, Rich. Let's call the police and get on with the bargaining attempts."

"There will be no police involvement. Don't you understand? This is a group of armed terrorists. I'm leaving now to see what I can do. Under no circumstances are you to call the police, unless you want Maya's blood on your hands!"

Rich stormed out of the office, barely noticing Josh, who ran to catch him. "Wait! I can help."

Rich turned to face the little man, who startled him by giving the Mayatan greeting. "Galactic Agent Josh at your service."

A smile of amazement lit Rich's face. "You new agents certainly use good cloaking devices." He then returned the greeting. "Galactic Agent Rich. Thanks for your offer. I'll take it."

Josh began, "Maya is in a tightly guarded, military camp that has been set up on the other side of Thunder Mountain."

"Is she all right?" Rich questioned.

"For now, yes."

"The military's involved?"

"I've done some checking on The Human Economics Movement," replied Josh. "It's run by a former three-star general, General George Gunnison, and his scientist girlfriend, Dr. Rosalyn Reichardt."

"What do they want?"

"Maya silenced. But beyond that, they want the *Owner's Manual* totally discredited."

"What are they afraid of?"

"Losing their economic position of superiority. As increasing numbers of the Earthlings remember their responsibility to the Earth, the economics of big business suffers from the environmental controls that are put into effect and from the more conscious buying habits of consumers. T.H.E.M. is a coalition, consisting of crooked politicians, right-wing military and religious extremists, and big business. They have the most to lose as the Earthlings have begun to remember their connection with their home planet."

"Okay. What else can you tell me?" Rich interrupted. "How desperate are they?"

"Very. In the last century, they represented the majority and needed no secret military force. Since the move toward global peace and peacemaking with the environment, their industries have suffered major losses. Many corporations that were built on greed and exploitation have been dying off. The remaining numbers have banded together in a desperate attempt to stop the flow of rapid change and empowerment that opposes the philosophy of putting humans first — at the expense of the natural resources and the animal world."

"What do you think they will do?"

"Well, Dr. Reichardt is intending to decode and reprogram Maya's brain, using her invention, the Brain Jammer."

"Can Maya survive this machine until we can rescue her?"

"I think so. If she can access her Galactic shield in time, she will be past this hurdle and on to the next."

"What next hurdle?" asked Rich.

"They're going to take what's left, after they think they have repatterned her brain, and publicly declare her a witch and a false messiah. Appealing to the fear-consciousness of the last century, they'll incite a large crowd to burn her for witchcraft!"

"Stop it! That cannot happen, Josh. How can we get her out of there?"

"We cannot. Mission *Owner's Manual* will be aborted if we intervene. Maya has chosen to accept this ordeal as her supreme test and the supreme test for Mission *Owner's Manual*."

Δ Δ Δ

Maya entered an altered state of consciousness, quickly accessing her harmonic frequency. She vaguely sensed electric current flowing through her body. Suddenly a man dressed in military uniform burst into the room, screaming, "Turn off your damn machine, Roz!"

Maya rode a surging jolt of current back to conscious awareness as the machine came to a halt. "What in the hell do you think you're doing, you bitch? I told you not to touch the prisoner until we've got her confession on tape. We can't afford to have her brain jammed before then!"

"It's okay, Generalissimo," Roz said calmly. "I'm just playing — no permanent damage yet, my dear."

"Unstrap her now, damn it! Do you want bruises on her arms for the entire world to see?"

"Okay! Okay! You're so totally left-brained, George — never have time for a little spontaneity!"

"Shut up and take care of her wrists!" The general turned to his aide, "Maintain an armed guard at all times. I can't trust this freaked-out scientist."

With an ice pack on each wrist, Maya was escorted to a conference room, where she was brought cold water and a hot meal. The meal consisted of beef stew, which she refused. The guard insisted, "You must eat. You look pale, and you've got a recording to make."

"No, thank you. I do not eat meat."

"You must eat this — General's orders!"

Just then the general stormed in. "For God's sake, get her some broccoli soup, if that's what she wants!"

The tall, thin, bald man faced her, his sinister eyes dark with hatred. "Now, Dr. Cristal, let's have a little talk. My name is General George Gunnison. You may call me General. My organization, The Human Economics Movement, has become an endangered species due to your *Owner's Manual* nonsense. With any tighter environmental controls, I'm afraid we'll all have to be eating vegetables instead of steak. There won't be enough money left to pay for real food or any land left to raise it on. We'll all be living in a national forest!"

"General, you are living in denial. Your only enemy is your fear of change."

"Come now, Dr. Cristal. Let's try to keep this a friendly discussion."

"Get to the point, General!"

"In exactly twelve hours, there will be a videotaped recording on all network news programs of Maya Cristal confessing that she is a witch and a false messiah. You will tell people to destroy their *Owner's Manuals* and forget all this self-empowerment and save-the-earth nonsense. The earth's not going to go anywhere. It's here for man's disposal. And if it does wear out, we'll just find a new and better planet! So let's get down to making that tape, what do you say?"

Maya looked directly into the General's cold, menacing eyes and calmly stated, "No."

"What do you mean, 'No?' We're talking about your life that's at stake here!"

"No. We are talking about the Earth's life and the life of her inhabitants, including you!"

"I don't need one of your goddamn ecolectures, just tell me yes or no, are you willing to die for this?"

"If necessary, yes. The *Owner's Manual* has opened the door of freedom of choice for millions of individuals who are returning balance and harmony to the Living Spaceship Earth. Nothing can stop the rising tide of empowerment — not you or your girlfriend, your organization, your political cohorts, or your entire army!"

"Think it over, Dr. Cristal. You're running out of

time." The General slammed the door, and Maya was escorted to her cell by the armed guard. She began to softly hum her five harmonic tones, over and over, slipping into Dreamtime awareness.

Δ Δ Δ

Maya's spirit resonated with the pure harmonic frequency that lifted her into a different space and time. She was walking in a beautiful garden, surrounded by many varieties of fruit trees. In the center of the garden one tree stood alone, surrounded by a deep pool. She looked into the pool, at first, seeing merely her reflection. Then the wind began to play with the surface of the water and her image started to transform. She heard a rustling near her feet, and the words, "Do not turn around, Sister. Be still while you experience my energy without resistance."

Maya saw herself reflected in the magic pool, only she had taken the form of a beautiful snake, a snake of many colors, shimmering, undulating in a rhythmic dance, a dance of ancient beauty. She moved to the sound of inner harmony, touching Earth and sky in her flowing movements. Shadows blended with rainbow light, filling her senses. This garden of nature, untouched, unspoiled, was home.

Suddenly the pool became dark, the dancing stopped, and the rainbow light was extinguished. With an agonizing cry she attempted to lift herself but was unable to move. "There are those whose hatred and fear call us the enemy," spoke the voice. "The only enemy is their raging fear."

Hot, searing wind began to blow — parching, destroying all greenness of life. Maya experienced emptiness, releasing cries of anguish and despair — why cannot this body lift from the ground? Cursed, cursed by anger and fear, chosen as the symbol of their darkness. Her body was being pulled tighter, skin stretched to its limit, past the breaking point, slowly, slowly going further into the pain. Suddenly the pool burst into flames. She entered the fire — hot, scorching blaze, brilliant orange-gold flames — in an explosion of light and sound.

This is breakthrough, release from the old skin, bringing back the ancient truths, the balance and harmony. Maya heard the song of one verse, a uni-verse, as she saw the image of the snake beyond the flames, dancing again in the rainbow light.

"You may step out of the flames now, Sister. Come, rest in the cool grass."

Maya felt herself moving out of a sheath of parched, dead skin. Her eyes met the gaze of a large snake. "You have experienced my curse. Now experience my healing." Maya tasted cool, refreshing fruit, the fruit of the tree, quenching her thirst.

"Because you have successfully transmuted my energy, you are aware that I represent a reflection of your changing self and of the Earthlings. They, like you, must have the courage to experience change without resistance. They, too, must come through the fire, releasing their fears. The only way out is always through."

Δ Δ Δ

When Maya returned to conscious awareness, she was lying on the cot in her darkened cell. Sensing the presence of familiar spirits nearby, she acknowledged them with love and reassurance. Then she drifted into a restful sleep.

She was awakened by a bright light shining in her eyes. "Wake up! Wake up! Are you ready to record yet?" demanded the General.

"No, never!"

"Then go to hell, you witch!"

A short time later, Maya was again disturbed, this time by Roz. "So you won't cooperate with the Generalissimo,

Princess? Maybe we can change that. He's given me permission to play with your brain, my dear."

Again, Paul strapped her into the chair, this time even more roughly than before. From the open door into the conference room, she could hear the General shouting, "I don't give a damn about what you require, Senator. The woman absolutely refuses to cooperate! Roz is our only hope...."

Maya released her conscious awareness, drifting on her harmonic tones just as a surge of electricity entered and passed through her body. After more shocks, the sound frequencies began to bombard her brain waves, attempting to attach themselves to her distant awareness, like torpedo missiles homing in on their target. Maya easily deflected each of these missiles with her harmonic shield. She became a silent observer to the operations performed on her brain, futile attempts to decode her Galactic memories, followed by reprogramming of T.H.E.M. propaganda. Roz became a madwoman at the controls, sending killer doses of hallucinogenic states through the electrical and sound frequencies.

"That's enough!" shouted the General. "Any normal human should be dead by now. Maybe what's left of her can still read a message into the camera. Liven up her face with some makeup."

Roz unstrapped the bands and removed the helmet, splashing cold water in Maya's face. "Now, Princess, how are we feeling?"

She opened her eyes to meet Roz's hatred with total acceptance. "I have never felt better, Doctor. You should try it yourself."

"Damn you! Are you going to record or not?"

"Now's your last chance!" threatened the General.

Maya felt only pity for their fear, as she matched their intensity, "No, no, no, never! I will never betray Gaia and Equadiety, regardless of your threats!"

"That's it! Notify the troops to prepare the site," the General ordered his aide.

"Such a waste of a good brain," muttered Roz. "You could have done T.H.E.M. so much good."

Maya was thrown into her cell by one of the guards. While she listened to the sounds of many footsteps outside the building, dragging of equipment, and orders being shouted, she contemplated the fear and hatred that consumed the General and his followers. These people are a dying breed, and my capture is their last hope for survival of their deranged way of thinking.

"Step aside for the camera crew," she heard the General order. "Are you sure you can get this edited for nationwide release by 10 o'clock?"

"Yes sir, General. For what your friends in Washington are paying, you could have this on the moon by 10 o'clock!"

Another bright light, and Maya was handcuffed and led out of her cell into the cool, night air and then up a path that she could sense was leading to Thunder Mountain. She heard the footsteps and voices of a large crowd behind her. With an abrupt order to halt, she was shoved into an area that had been cleared in the middle of the forest. A large tree in the center of the clearing remained untouched. One of the guards attached a chain and ropes to her handcuffs, tying her to the tree. Then soldiers piled small branches around her feet.

Maya looked fearlessly at the gathering. The General, Roz, and Paul were in the front of the crowd, lighting torches. Others in military uniform, and some in business suits also had torches. There were even families with young children. She heard a baby crying and sent it thoughts of love and assurance.

The eyes staring at her reflected hatred and fear, along with the excitement of soldiers hungry for battle. As torches were passed among the crowd, Maya spoke boldly, "Allow my words to enter your hearts. What you fear is change — change from what you have learned from generations of misdirected power and self-serving greed. But this change should not be feared. It should be welcomed as a return to balance and harmony with our true mother — Mother Earth — Gaia, the living, breathing planet we call home. Your separation from the Earth is an illusion, based on lies. Awaken to truth — remember your noble spirit — love plus understanding is the answer, not hate and fear. Release your bond of fear and follow the path of freedom — the path of the heart ..."

"Silence the witch, the false prophet of doom!" The General rushed forward first, screaming obscenities, as he ignited the branches and the hem of Maya's robe. Roz followed, and then the crowd pressed in, quickly throwing their torches on the blaze, chanting, "Death to the witch, death from T.H.E.M. to you!"

Maya began humming her harmonic tones, first softly, then louder and louder as the flames rose around her. Then she heard a voice whispering, "It is I, Maya, the Tree of Understanding. You are surrounded by friends."

Beginning to float on her harmonic frequency, she could distinguish forms moving among the flames. "Do not resist, dear Sister," came the haunting cry of the whale. "Our Living Spaceship Earth will be saved. Your Truth is a healing force."

"It seems upside down," whispered a vampire bat, "but they are the ones in chains, not you."

"Only cowards resort to acts of aggression and violence," communicated the jaguar.

Maya looked down at the chains on her wrists. They took on the appearance of writhing serpents, coiling and uncoiling around her. She released herself to the protection of her Galactic shield and her five harmonic tones.

As the explosive heat spread through her body, her skin pulled tighter and tighter. Then she heard the howl of the wolf, Cyruse, exploding into a cry of triumph as she carried Maya on her back through the tree tops, a stream of flames trailing behind them.

Δ Δ Δ

"Good evening, this is Margaret Lemonde. The world has lost a champion, and we at the *STAR* Network have lost a friend. Tonight's top story records the apparent assassination, this evening, of Dr. Maya Cristal, host of the highly acclaimed program, 'High Performance Adventure.'

"Dr. Cristal was kidnapped last night while leaving the *STAR* studios. The Human Economics Movement has taken responsibility for the kidnapping in a note sent to the producer of 'High Performance Adventure,' Rich Land. The demand made by T.H.E.M. was for Dr. Cristal to confess to being a witch and a false messiah. A videotape of the bizarre assassination was delivered to our station by a courier for their organization. That tape is coming up next, followed by interviews with members of the crowd, conducted by Ginny Donovan, of our news staff, who arrived at the scene just after the apparent assassination of Dr. Cristal. Here now is that videotape."

"I am General George Gunnison, President of The Human Economics Movement. What you are about to see is an important step in the development of mankind. The false messiah and witch, Maya Cristal, is no more. She had set herself up to oppose the welfare of man, even the survival of life as we know and cherish it.

"The Human Economics Movement believes in the God-given superiority of man over all other species. We believe it is our right to have dominion over the land, the air, and the sea, and to use all resources for our human benefit. Because of our natural superiority, mankind was chosen to rule and subdue the earth.

"Toward the end of the 20th Century, numerous grassroots movements began to spread a false gospel of equality for all species, campaigning for environmental controls, inhibiting the fair growth of human economics. Now the 21st Century has brought the impostor, Maya Cristal, brainwashing these misguided souls into a worldwide movement to strip mankind of our God-given superiority. This impostor had to be silenced before we were all forced to live like animals instead of men.

"Realizing her sins and her folly, Dr. Cristal agreed to serve as a human sacrifice so that order may be returned to the earth. Here now is the film coverage of her demise.

"You can see the flames beginning to rise around Dr. Cristal. As the branches around her begin to blaze, she utters a cry of anguish and collapses ..."

Margaret Lemonde: "You notice that there were major edits toward the end of that clip. Here now is the footage filmed by our own reporter, Ginny Donovan."

"This is Ginny Donovan. I arrived at the scene immediately after the apparent assassination of Dr. Maya Cristal. Here are some reports from members of the crowd."

Crowd Member #1: "This is the strangest thing I've ever witnessed. I don't understand what happened, but I believe she's alive. I saw shadows of animal figures surrounding her in the flames. I think maybe she's an angel instead of a witch."

Crowd Member #2: "No way, man! That witch is dead. Some of her followers must have sneaked in during the storm and taken her remains for burial. I saw her burning alive in there."

Crowd Member #3: "The storm was so sudden and violent, and the fire was extinguished so quickly. It seemed like magic to me!"

Crowd Member #4: "Look at those chains. They're melted. No human could survive that blaze. She's dead, man!"

Ginny Donovan: "But what about the tree? Why is it untouched, and where are the remains of Dr. Cristal?"

Crowd Member #4: "Beats me. I'm getting out of here. This is too weird!"

Crowd Member #5: "I saw Maya Cristal on the back of a huge animal, pure white, howling in the flames. Then, in a flash, they were up in the air, high above our heads. I saw a trail of fire behind them as they took off like a comet through the sky."

Crowd Member #6: "This woman's crazy. She's suffering from smoke inhalation."

Ginny Donovan: "Where is Maya Cristal? Is she dead or alive? If she is alive, the question on all our minds is 'Who is she, really?' This is Ginny Donovan, with the *STAR* Network. Now back to Margaret Lemonde with the 10 o'clock report."

Margaret Lemonde: "Just moments ago, the FBI arrived at the scene of the apparent assassination of Dr. Maya Cristal. A warrant has been issued for the arrest of General Gunnison and his accomplice, Dr. Rosalyn Reichardt. An investigation is under way into The Human Economics Movement. Their headquarters in Washington, D.C. is being searched for evidence of criminal intent. An unidentified source has named a prominent U.S. senator as an active member of the coalition. Stay tuned for further developments."

Δ Δ Δ

The fiery explosion of Maya and Cyruse had caused a sudden violent storm to drench the crowd and the fire. Jagged bolts of lightning from a cloudless sky had filled the air, along with a deafening, thunderous roar, accompanied by a raging wind.

Moving rapidly through the darkness, vaulting into a star-filled sky, and then into warm, golden sunlight, Maya and Cyruse traveled far from the scene, arriving in a distant land. They were greeted by an aqua blue sky, trees with heart-shaped leaves, and flowers that burst into bloom as they approached. The winding road led to a river that glowed with a mysterious light. As they reached the shore, soft grass and then warm sand caressed Maya's bare feet. She said aloud, "What sort of magical river could this be?"

"I am called Jewel River," answered a musical voice. "Come, experience my healing treasures." It was truly a river of jewels. Shimmering, clear water danced with millions of gemstones and crystals — rose quartz, blue topaz, turquoise, amethysts, emeralds, rubies, sapphires, opals and many, many more.

Maya stepped into the water, letting herself flow gently with the current. The gems' polished surfaces brushed against her body, sending rainbows of color throughout her senses. She reached into the water and cupped handfuls of the healing stones, immersing herself in their subtle energies. What exquisite beauty each reflects in the brilliant sunlight, she thought.

A ribbon of light encircled Maya as she dove into the sparkling water. One by one, her five spirit tones greeted her, blending in a harmony that flowed through her in a baptism of light and sound. Allowing herself to sink deeper and deeper into the water, she released conscious awareness, and was swept into the center of the river. She became a part of its potent force, rushing onward with surging power.

River of life — of renewal — we are birthing a new reality. Now is the time to accept our power and to remember our bond with the Living Spaceship Earth. Awareness — wisdom is remembering, becoming conscious of our connection to the divine — accepting our divinity. Releasing doubt and fear, guilt and obedience ... choosing freedom, responsibility, transformation — the path of the heart.

Once again, Maya transformed into the purest of crystals — a representation of Truth — and was washed ashore in a beautiful wooded park. Sparkling in the sunlight, she attracted the attention of a young woman and her little boy. "Look, Ethan," the woman said. "What a magical toy I've found for you. Would you like to take it home?"

The little boy stared intently at the crystal and shook his head, "No, Mama. It doesn't want to come home with us. It doesn't belong to us. It belongs to everyone."

"You're right, son," his mother replied, tears filling her eyes as she looked at the radiant face of her child. "Where did you get such wisdom, Ethan?"

"I think I remembered it, Mama."

Chapter 26

The Church

Maya was greeted by Rich as she slipped in the side entrance of the television station. "I'm so glad to see you, Maya! You have been on my mind constantly!"

"Thank you, Rich. I sensed your presence frequently during the past week."

"Thanks for your call filling me in on all the details of your ordeal. I wish we had more time to talk — maybe after the show... I'm glad you're here early. There are about a dozen women who want to meet with you in the conference room before the show. I forgot to tell you about it before now, but the meeting has been arranged for over a week. I don't know what they want. They are twelve leaders from every aspect of business, government and education. There's even a high official from the Ecumenical Council."

"Rich, you know that I am a very private person. Please do not schedule meetings for me in the future. What is their agenda?"

"I'm not certain, but I believe they are sincere in their zeal for your work. You really need to talk to them yourself. I'll walk with you to the conference room."

As Maya and Rich entered the conference room in silence, the twelve women rose to their feet in unison. Maya circled the room, introducing herself to each of the women. The leader of the group was Carole Light, president of Energy Research Laboratories, Inc. Carole quickly dismissed Rich by saying, "Rich, we appreciate your arranging this meeting of women only."

He smiled an acknowledgement and left the room, closing the door behind him.

"Maya, we knew you would return! Our whole group was in a panic for a while, but I kept saying, 'She'll be back. She'll be back,'" Carole began.

"Thank you for your concern. Now please tell me your purpose in requesting this meeting," Maya stated firmly.

"We have struggled as to how to approach you with our request. All of us are experts in our chosen fields. Most are outspoken leaders in both community and world affairs. In order to eliminate communication errors, I would like to read our statement of intent."

"Please proceed."

"'We, the original twelve members of the Cristal Council, do hereby declare our steadfast beliefs:

"1) Maya Cristal is the first female messiah sent to correct the ills of our troubled world. Male messiahs have been sent throughout time, and their missions have always resulted in male-dominated, dictatorial organizations, which enslave women, children, and minorities. As women, we have bought into belief systems that kept us in bondage by telling us what to do, what to believe, and how to act. These commandments are like mental and spiritual chains, robbing us of our ability to use our *Owner's Manuals* for our brains. We then enslave our children by programming them with the same limiting beliefs.

"We have been programmed that if we do not follow the male-created dogma, we will burn in a future hell. These organizations thus rob our past and our present, and damn our future by demanding strict obedience to a rigid belief system. We suffer from guilt and rejection if we attempt to escape. There is only one hope, and that hope is through the perfect spiritual organization which we have chosen to call the Cristal Clear Church.

"2) We place no blame on past messiahs. Their intentions were pure, and if followed with perfect love, would have led to mental and spiritual freedom for all.

"3) We release from blame the past male-dominated organizations, their leaders, and followers. They did what they thought was right. They did not have *Owner's Manuals* for their brains.

"4) Women must be the ones to organize this new Church, since we were not directly involved with the prior attempts at religious perfection. Women will honor the integrity of all without enslaving anyone under a rigid system.

"5) Dr. Maya Cristal will be the head of the Church and will train twelve women to follow in her path. These twelve will each train twelve. These 144 will each train twelve until every woman in the world will be a practitioner of the *Owner's Manual* concept.

"6) The Cristal Clear Church will meet once a week (on Sunday since our society accepts that custom). This meeting will serve to reinforce the group's acceptance, plus serve to educate new members.

"7) Dr. Maya Cristal will deliver a weekly message via closed circuit TV to all Cristal Clear Church facilities. Donations will finance the organization's present liabilities, plus fund future growth. Outreach programs will be organized for other countries of the world.

"8) Dr. Maya Cristal will have the exclusive right to name her successor. Future heads of the Cristal Clear Church will be selected by the twelve members of the Cristal Council. Cristal Council members serve for life and are replaced by the vote of existing members of the Council.

"9) Policies, procedures, official publications, and

recruiting materials will be written and/or approved by the Cristal Council, with the total veto power of Dr. Maya Cristal or her successor.

"10) The Cristal Clear Church will be in place and fully functional on or before one year from today's date.

"This document was written and approved by the Cristal Council of the Cristal Clear Church of America.

"Maya, as you can easily see, we intend to create the perfect spiritual organization. Will you accept this honor and assist us in making our dream a reality?"

Maya responded, "Thank you for your offer. I know you mean well. I suggest another path to your outcome of spiritual freedom.

"First, I am not your messiah. You must be your own messiah. Do not organize another religion, another church, another temple. To encapsulate TRUTH into religious dogma, no matter how pure the intent, would be repeating the mistakes of the past. Accept your personal power balanced with love, and the chains of dogma will have no control over you.

"Do not think of yourselves as women separate from men. Men are not your enemy. They are your partners. Your spirit is neither female nor male. Until you learn to be in partnership with your feminine and masculine energy, then you are only half a person.

"Your Cristal Clear Church is an organization that would eventually rob its members of their personal freedom, as have all organizations in the past. Personal power can never come from an organization, no matter how pure its intent.

"There will be no physical Cristal Clear Church. You have a question?"

"Yes," Carole replied. "I'm very disappointed but not surprised by your response. How can we help, Maya? We know your *Owner's Manual* concept is transforming the world."

"Simply live your life so that no one can misunderstand your message. Do not begin by trying to change the world. Begin by changing yourself, your world."

Maya remained for a few moments in the silent room. The women looked at her with respect and understanding.

Δ Δ Δ

Rich stopped Maya on her way to her office. "What was that all about?"

"Pure spirit brought to Earth has always been misunderstood — condemned as the Devil by some — worshiped by others. Pure spirit simply is. Do you understand, Rich?"

"Yes, Maya. I understand. I wish that I ... that you ... I'll see you on the set."

Chapter 27

The Transformation Adventure

"**G**ood evening. My name is Rich Land, producer of 'High Performance Adventure.' Last week we announced on our 10 o'clock news here at the *STAR* Network that Dr. Maya Cristal was the apparent victim of assassination. The Human Economics Movement, T.H.E.M., took credit for her kidnapping and subsequent assassination. Since our first announcement, there has been an investigation into this coalition, headed by General George Gunnison and his accomplice, Dr. Rosalyn Reichardt. They have been arrested and charged with kidnapping, assault, and murder.

"In related developments, the recent suicide of Senator Sam Byrnstein from New York has been linked to his association with T.H.E.M. William McGuffee, head of HUD, and long-time friend and associate of General Gunnison, has been missing from his home in Washington for three days. An unidentified source reported seeing a man matching his description boarding a plane for Baghdad two days ago. Approximately two thousand members of T.H.E.M. have officially resigned from the organization and demanded its immediate dissolution.

"It is my pleasure to announce that Dr. Maya Cristal is alive and in perfect health! After taking a few days of rest from her ordeal, she has arrived at the studio and will be on the set in a few moments. She will make a short statement and will answer questions from the audience before beginning tonight's 'High Performance Adventure.' But first, here is the film clip of the attempt on her life."

The studio monitor flashed scenes of the restless crowd around an enormous tree, illuminated with floodlights. The video was frequently disrupted by lighting problems, pushing and shoving of the crowd, and by apparent editing of the tape.

Next came the blurred image of Maya, dressed in a flowing, white robe, being led through the crowd to the execution tree. Ropes and chains quickly secured her, while small branches were piled around her. A close-up showed Maya's face as she spoke passionately to the crowd, although her words were unintelligible, drowned by the shouts of the onlookers.

The chanting of "Death to the witch" could be heard, as torches ignited the branches around Maya. What followed was a blur of disorganized camera work, obvious film cuts, and complete hysteria. Maya appeared to be engulfed by flames, but slow motion indicated no sign of fear or pain. Shadowy figures resembling a whale, giant vampire bats, a jaguar, and snakes appeared in the flames with her. Finally the unmistakable form of a gigantic wolf appeared, and with an unearthly howl, Maya and the wolf exploded into the sky, trailing a comet's burst of fire.

Simultaneously, there was a deafening sound of thunder, followed by torrents of rain from a star-filled sky. Steam and smoke filled the screen as the fire was quickly extinguished by the sudden downpour. When the screen cleared, the drenched crowd was moving about in frantic disarray. Some ran from the scene in panic. Others knelt in awe, appearing to be praying for forgiveness. General Gunnison and Dr. Reichardt could be seen, hurrying from the area with a military escort.

Panic and reverence were mixed in a tossed salad of human emotions. The studio monitor went black in an abrupt ending, leaving the audience in stunned silence. Rich looked toward the stage curtains and announced, "Here she is now. Please welcome Dr. Maya Cristal!"

The studio audience rose to their feet in a standing ovation. The cheering stopped abruptly as Maya began to speak. *"Good evening, everyone. Thank you for your love and concern.*

"The past week has been an interesting and deeply moving experience. The reports of my kidnapping and torture are correct, with the obvious exception of my assassination. I am requesting that the charges be dropped against General George Gunnison and Dr. Rosalyn Reichardt, and any other member of T.H.E.M., and I am requesting their immediate release. Because of their unsuccessful attempt to assassinate me, they and their coalition, T.H.E.M., have been exposed and rendered powerless.

"There is not enough time to give you all the details of this experience. I was able to use the full power of mind and spirit to negate the forces used against me. I offered no physical resistance, and I felt no fear. When you have fully developed your Owner's Manual for your brain, you will understand completely. I will accept a few questions before we begin our scheduled program, the 'Transformation Adventure.'"

Audience Members #1, 2, and 3: "Maya, Maya ... what happened?"

"One question at a time, please. What did you see happening?"

Audience Member #1: "What I just viewed was very confusing to me. It appeared as though you simply exploded into the sky on the back of a huge wolf. What happened? How did you do that?"

"Do you believe that is what happened?"

Audience Member #1: "Yes ... yes, I do. I don't know how you did it, but I know that's what happened."

"If you believe it, then that is what happened. Your perception equals your reality. Do not resist what your heart has led you to believe."

Audience Member #2: "I saw you explode in a ball of fire! You must have been dead. You transcended death!"

"Then that is what happened. Your perception equals your reality."

Audience Member #3: "I saw the shapes of animals in the flames with you. You must be able to communicate with the spirit world."

"Then that is what happened. Your perception equals your reality."

Audience Member #4: "How did you escape without any burns? It's not humanly possible to survive such an ordeal, let alone look as if nothing happened! Have you had a medical examination — I mean, have the doctors examined you, because I think you must be from another planet or something. I know you can't possibly be human, unless that was trick photography! I'm not a spiritual person, but what I just saw was the most spiritual experience I've ever had. I'm only human, you know, so this is hard for me to accept."

"The error most people make is to believe that we are human beings having a spiritual experience. Instead, we are spiritual beings having a human experience. I repeat, we are all spiritual beings having a human experience."

Audience Member #5: "Can you tell us why you have requested the release of these criminals? They're a threat to society!"

"There is no punishment equal to the hell they have created for themselves. I am in no danger from them, and neither is anyone else. Because their vehicle for hatred and greed has been destroyed, they are harmless to everyone but themselves. My purpose, my mission is not to punish, but to set people free — all people."

Audience Member #6: "What did they do to you?"

"The news reports have dealt with my kidnapping and torture, and also with the attempt to burn me to death. There was no damage because I was totally protected from harm."

Audience Member #7: "I think you were sent by the Devil to tempt people to convert to your philosophy."

"Then to you, that is what I am. Whatever we see in another is always a mirror of our true selves. Your perception equals your reality."

Audience Member #8: "How could someone who has done so much good be of the Devil? I'm tired of such narrow-minded, fear-based accusations! I believe that Maya Cristal is sent from someplace beyond this world, to show us the perfect example of using our *Owner's Manuals.* I truly believe that I, too, can develop the ability to use my mind and spirit to the point that I can overcome physical or mental danger, and live a life of peace, love, and understanding."

"Then that is true for you. Your perception equals your reality.

"Thank you for your questions.

"We are living in a time of the most rapid transformation in the history of the Planet Earth. Tonight we will be dealing with breakthrough and change in the 'Transformation Adventure.' Our first guest has a Ph.D. in psychology and change management. Author of numerous books, and father of two children, he is much in demand as a professional speaker and seminar leader. Please welcome Dr. Leo Townsend."

"I'm so glad you are safe and sound, Maya. I'm an avid believer in the Brainware you are helping people to develop for their *Owner's Manuals.*"

"*Thank you, Leo. I have been looking forward to meeting you because of your leadership in the return to balance within organizations. What is the most dramatic transformation occurring at this time?*"

"Wow! I was hoping you'd ask me that question! It's partnership — from individual to global. Partnership is transforming our family systems, the way we raise and educate our children, our relationships, our workplace, our government, and our attitude and actions toward our planet."

"*I love your passion for this subject! Tell us more.*"

"Where should I start? We're experiencing the end of a long history of male domination in every aspect of society from families to religion — a male dominance that caused co-dependence and addictive behaviors. After all, it's not feminine energy that has gotten us into trouble. We haven't suffered from burdensome amounts of nurturance and empathy. Rather, intolerance, greed, aggression, war, exploitation of people, and especially exploitation of our planetary resources are all the result of male dominance. I'm not saying all evils have been caused by men — for too many years women cooperated with male dominance — it's masculine energy — the masculine energy in both men and women that has been out of balance for thousands of years.

"I believe we've entered a new paradigm of partnership which began with self-transformation — change always begins with the individual. We're entering a time of widespread acceptance by individuals of their dual feminine and masculine nature. As we return ourselves to balance, we can welcome partnership relationships."

"*How is the role of women transforming?*"

"The rising status of women — long overdue — is

beginning to move us closer to equality of jobs, pay, property ownership, and most of all, respect. The nurturing feminine energy with its creativity and innovation is transforming the workplace through right-brain enhancement."

"How is that happening?"

"The giant, left-brained, heartless corporations of the past have shrunk — or died and been reborn as smaller, nurturing, supportive, family-type organizations. The new workplace encourages risk taking and creativity. It's a place of great flexibility — a place where individuals are empowered to find balance and fulfillment in their careers."

"How are men handling this transformation?"

"The paradigm shift from male dominance to partnership is challenging, to say the least, and many men are still resisting. Those of us who have welcomed the transformation are relaxing into an acceptance of our open, trusting, and nurturing natures. An example of this is the widespread practice of men taking a paternity leave of six weeks to three months for the birth of their children. I did this with my second child, Melody, and wow! What a bond we have!"

"What other changes are occurring in child raising?"

"The education system is beginning to transform to a more wholebrained approach. Children are being taught self-esteem, and there is less programming of fear and guilt. The research has proven that children who value themselves and others are far less likely to be susceptible to dysfunctional behaviors such as drugs, alcohol, and other addictions that have plagued our youth and our society.

"You know, we had it all wrong at the end of the last century when we declared war on drugs. That obviously was a costly, national disaster. War is never a remedy because it's an unbalanced, aggressive, left-brained approach. We've finally discovered that empowerment is the answer. Children who are taught self-esteem and personal power in a nurturing, supportive environment don't need to get involved in addictive, co-dependent behaviors to feel important.

"Co-dependence used to thrive in families which supported each other's addictions, and in the military and in religious organizations which demanded blind obedience. These organizations fostered co-dependence by teaching us to give our power away to the church, the government, the corporation, to family, friends, the media, peers, and the list goes on. We were taught that it was noble to sacrifice ourselves. Well that's masochistic! There needs to be a balance between self and others, true, but that comes about when we use our personal power with integrity."

"What governmental changes exemplify partnership?"

"That's been the slowest area of transformation. The candidacy of Senator Sheril Wilkinson for president — number one in the Gallup Polls — is the most dramatic change ... listen to that applause. Yes! It's about time, isn't it?

"Globally, the acceptance of peace has been the result of a return to a more balanced society. As men have released their need to play war games, the military is beginning to re-form as a corps of men and women dedicated to solving the problems of world hunger, poverty, and making peace with the environment. We're beginning to show dramatic changes as we move toward restoring ecobalance because we're transforming our attitude from ownership of the Earth to partnership with our living Earth home.

"Because we no longer are investing billions of tax dollars in the technology of war and destruction, our quality of life is increasing with lower taxes and far greater government spending for education, the arts, and most important, the environment."

"I commend you for your passionate involvement in the return to balance, Leo. Who was your role model?"

"My father is a beautiful balance of feminine nurturing and masculine results orientation. From him I learned that I alone am responsible for what I choose to create in my life. If we will choose to build a healthy relationship with ourselves — one based on a balance of our feminine and masculine natures — then we will be able to have healthy partnership relationships with others, and we will welcome transformation instead of resisting it."

"Thank you, Leo, for your insight into the exciting transformation that is occurring. Now we have some questions from our audience."

Audience Member #9: "I can't believe what I heard you say about religion! What do you mean that it's disempowering? You know that our society was built on religion, on the Ten Commandments, and God's law. If we don't have God in our lives, what hope do we have?"

Leo: "I would like to clarify that. I certainly believe in the importance of a spiritual life, and for many people, God represents their spirituality. However, if we end up worshiping the rules, instead of God, or our idea of God, we become dependent on an organization to validate us, and we lose sight of our own power as spiritual human beings.

"Religion allows us to be comfortable by living in a box that says we are Methodist, Catholic, Buddhist, or whatever. And we have our lives defined by our box called our religion, our nationality, political affiliation, and the list goes on. In order to be able to welcome the changes we face on a daily basis, we must get out of our comfortable little boxes called our belief systems. If Christ had accepted his box, and just remained a carpenter in a small village, his work and words would be unknown today."

Audience Member #10: "But I'm comfortable in my comfort zone. I don't want to change."

Leo: "Change is inevitable — growth is optional."

Audience Member #11: "I work in a small company with sixteen employees, and you're right, it's like a family. One person acts like my dad, and then there's Mom, Sis, uncles, aunts and bratty kids. I would love to see more left-brained, business logic. I don't want to be smothered with all this corporate family nonsense."

Leo: "What is your job?"

Audience Member #11: "Cost accounting and production scheduling."

Leo: "What would you like to be doing?"

Audience Member #11: "Oh, sales or personnel ..."

Leo: "Most people will enjoy the corporate family if they are in the position that fulfills their potential. I suggest that you choose to transfer to a position that suits you."

"Thank you, Leo, for being a passionate example of balance in action."

"Thank you, Maya, for this opportunity. It is very special to be in your presence."

"Every moment is special, Leo.

"Our next guest is a woman who has learned to deal with, even welcome transformation. She recently retired from her position as president of a bank holding company in the Midwest. Please welcome Connie Philips."

"Hello, Maya, Leo. I've been looking forward to meeting you, Maya."

"Thank you, Connie. Please tell us your background."

"Well, I grew up in a small town in Arkansas, the daughter of an alcoholic father and an enabler mother — we were an extremely dysfunctional, co-dependent family. When I was sixteen, I fell in love with my ex-husband — I'll call him John. I was looking for a way out of my unhappiness."

"What happened?"

"After we were married and had our son, my husband started beating me. I had always known he was aggressive, but I had no idea he was violent."

"He gave no signs of this tendency when you were dating?"

"No, he was jealous and possessive, but nothing more."

"What did you do about the beatings?"

"I left him many times, but I would go back, because I was afraid he would hunt me down and kill me."

"We have frequently mentioned on this program that everyone and everything in our lives is a mirror for us. How was your former husband a mirror for you?"

"I've thought a lot about that. First of all, my marriage was a mirror of society. All the songs, the movies, all of society's expectations for a woman were that she would get married and have children and live happily ever after. So, I accepted that programming and lived out the typical expectations, except for the happily ever after part.

"I've really looked at how the mirror principle applied to my relationship with John — and how I managed to stay with him for twelve years. He had no respect for himself or for women, and I guess I had lost my self-respect. Also, I used to become quite brutal and fight back when he beat me."

"How did you find the courage to leave him?"

"I just did it. I took my son and ran away to a small town in Texas. I completely rebuilt my life. I went to college and began my career in banking."

"How did you deal with the anger and bitterness you must have felt?"

"I've accepted that everything in my life is there to teach me lessons I need to learn. One day a co-worker asked me why I was so impatient and bitter. That question helped me realize that I had wasted far too much energy on my anger. I used to lie awake at night scheming how I could get even with John. How absurd! The only person I was hurting was myself.

"One thing that was a big help was to repeat positive affirmations to myself, over and over, especially as I was drifting off to sleep. I would say, 'I forgive myself. I forgive John. I am a loving person. I deserve to be a loving person. I am powerful. I deserve to be powerful,' and the list went on. I used to have nightmares about John finding me and about our fights. I knew that I had released my hatred when I stopped having the nightmares. One night I dreamed about him, and we were friends. It was after that dream that I felt a complete release from all my anger and bitterness."

"Do you believe that you were victimized by society's expectations and by John?"

"No. My opinion is that there are no victims — only volunteers. I gave away my power to my family and to John. When I could face that I was in a bad relationship because of the choices I had made, I was able to reclaim my power. That's what it's all about — life is a series of choices, and we have to be willing to take responsibility for the consequences of those choices."

"Have you remarried?"

"Yes, I have a wonderful, nurturing husband, and his three daughters, along with my son. Of course, the children are grown now, with families of their own. Larry and I are extremely happy together. He complements me by mirroring aspects of myself that I'd forgotten were there. He's helped me to remember that I'm a powerful person and to be comfortable with who I am. Larry and I are partners in an interdependent relationship which is like a beautiful dance."

"What would you like to say about the transformation of women?"

"That's one of my favorite subjects! I've seen women taking quantum leaps recently — from the position of victim to claiming a position of power. We've had to overcome many self-imposed barriers, such as our fear of change and our enabling personalities that created the need to please everyone, to be nice and agreeable under impossible circumstances without standing up for ourselves. Other barriers have been our perfectionism, our 'trying harder,' self-discounting, and the big 'O' for obedience to others' expectations and demands."

"How are women transforming themselves?"

"We've remembered that our true power lies in accepting both our feminine and masculine sides. Most of us went through a period of intense denial of our feminine selves, hating men, while trying our best to emulate them, to the point of dressing in pinstripe suits with noxious, little silk bow ties! We became imitation men, trying to force our way into the board room. Well, it didn't work. All we got was a lot of Type A behavior, with its stress-related health problems, and a lot of isolation from ourselves, the men we were jealous of, and our sisters. We had to get back in balance."

"What is causing the return to balance?"

"It's because we're valuing nurturing qualities in the workplace — that's exactly the paradigm shift Leo was describing. In fact, partnership in the business world is a part of that shift — the true partnership of interdependence. It's a respect for ourselves, as both men and women recognize that we are all one — more similar than we are different — we just happen to be living in different bodies."

"What about the changes men are experiencing?"

"A big part of the transformation of women is the acceptance by men of their nurturing qualities. And it is equally important that women are accepting these qualities in men. The macho man is a dinosaur. Men are going through a metamorphosis in learning to accept their feminine side, in nurturing their families and co-workers. They are having to learn to take equal responsibility for raising children, cleaning, cooking, and so on. There's still some imbalance in that men may have equal responsibility in the home, but it's often the woman who retains emotional responsibility by having to remind her partner to get the chores done, or by not letting go of the emotional responsibilities that used to be strictly hers. Women and men still have a lot to learn about balance, but we've come a great distance toward co-creating partnerships in our personal and business lives. And it had to begin by being in partnership with ourselves, by remembering our true power."

"You have been highly successful in the business world. What have you learned?"

"I've had it all — the private jet, fancy cars, beautiful homes, exotic vacations, all the material possessions. My greatest joy has been that I've learned how to be. All the successes were exciting — even some of the struggles — but they are not the real me. My greatest lesson has been to live in the moment, to accept myself and everything around me as perfect in each moment — that's where I am now.

"I also want to say that I recognize you, Maya, as an advanced soul who fully accepts her power. You are a mirror of the perfection in each of us, and I thank you for your glowing light which is helping to transform many lives."

"Thank you, Connie. Your transformation is an inspiration."

Audience Member #12: "I hesitate to ask this question because I'm proud of the strides women are making in transforming from the demeaning roles of cook, maid, and general subservient helpmate of men. Anyway, my question is, Why do so many men seem to feel emasculated as women take on more and more jobs that were formerly 'male only' positions? Whenever I hear some guy complaining about having to look after the kids, cook his own meals, wash his own clothes, or iron his own shirts, while his wife is away on some business trip, I notice that his divorce takes place within a year or so. Are women upsetting a somewhat natural balance of work within a marriage?"

Connie: "My mother would agree with you. She was perfectly happy doing what was considered 'woman's work,' while my dad mowed the lawn, washed the car, handled all the home repairs, did the taxes, and took out the trash. The fact remains, our society will not revert back to the 'good old days.'

"Let's examine the real issue here. Men, in general, like to feel superior because they are often physically stronger than we are. Mentally and spiritually, we are their equals. If a man chooses to feel emasculated by washing clothes or changing a diaper, then as Maya says, 'His perception equals his reality.' It's not women's responsibility to feed the ego of men any more than it's men's responsibility to keep women on a pedestal mentally, and barefoot and pregnant physically. My suggestion is for men to accept reality and be willing to accept women as equal partners. Enlightened men have already joined us. The past is not a very good place to live."

"Thank you, Connie. I celebrate your understanding of how to be.

"Our next guest is a healer who is working to facilitate transformation on an individual and planetary level. Please welcome Sierra Moreno."

"Good evening. I salute your Goddess energy, Maya. Your presence on the Earth plane has brought about much transformation."

"Thank you, Sierra. How did you decide to follow the

medicine path, since you are not a Native American?"

"Actually the path found me. For a long time I had been very interested in natural healing. Then I developed a fascination for medicinal plants. Soon I was being invited to attend childbirths, and from there, I became a practicing midwife.

"I've come through much personal transformation. I began my adult life in a far different field — the field of modeling and acting. I grew up in Hollywood and used to hang around motion picture sets. One day an agent asked me to audition for a commercial. I got the job and soon began doing television and print modeling. Then I got some small parts in a couple of movies. I was considering going to acting school when I met some friends who changed my life.

"They were folk singers and environmental activists who were demonstrating and lobbying for environmental issues. They had just spent several weeks helping to clean up a wildlife sanctuary after an oil spill along the California coast. I looked at my life, with its plastic beauty, and all the glamour, and I looked at their passionate involvement in changing the world, and I quit. I just walked away from my blossoming career and began to travel with them in their remodeled bus. We took on federal and state agencies, demonstrating, writing letters, distributing pamphlets, and educating people about solutions for a return to balance with Mother Earth.

"One day we stopped to visit an American Indian reservation in New Mexico. There I met the medicine woman who eventually became my teacher in learning the ways of the ancients."

"Will you explain why the ancient ways are so important?"

"The ancient ones followed the path of the heart. They understood the importance of balancing the spirit, mind, and body. And they knew how to listen to the wisdom of Mother Earth. They learned from the sun, the moon, the wind, the mountains, the trees, and all the animals, whom they considered our brothers and sisters. They knew the role of each plant in the forest and how it could be used for nourishment and healing. The ways of native peoples have been to live in harmony and balance, adapting themselves to Mother Earth. Non-native peoples have adapted nature to fit their needs, acting from a position of ownership of the Earth and committing crimes against our sacred land.

"Our modern society has become totally separated from the land and its wisdom — which means we have become separated from our spiritual selves — resulting in disharmony, and disease. The environmental crisis is a mirror of the inner spiritual crisis. That's why it is imperative that we heal ourselves before we can heal the planet."

"How do you teach people to heal themselves?"

"I facilitate workshops in which people confront their spiritual selves and their true purpose. We explore belief systems and how they have caused us to stay stuck and live in denial, which results in physical and emotional disease. Then we focus on a return to personal balance through the use of ritual and ceremony, which bonds participants to the Earth and helps them to discover their higher purpose."

"How did your family accept your decision to follow this path?"

"Not well, at first. My parents are extremely conservative, and they are also very devout Christians. They were shocked when I began modeling and acting because they believed this career would lead me into evil. When I told them of my new spiritual understanding and of my embracing the healing arts, they were brokenhearted. They said that they could never again respect me, and that I should crawl on my knees back to

God, begging forgiveness."

"How did you deal with their rejection?"

"In the beginning, I chose to experience a lot of negative emotions and to buy into their guilt trip. As I realized that we are not in this world to live up to others' expectations, I chose to release my fear of their wrath and my guilt over disappointing them. I have accepted the responsibility of healing and nurturing myself, and as I have done so, they have begun to understand that I'm doing what is right for me. They, too, are learning the importance of tolerance and acceptance, and our relationship is beginning to grow strong again.

"It used to be a compulsion for me to make people happy and fulfill their expectations. I was brought up in a co-dependent home, and so I became an enabler — someone who cooperates with others' addictions."

"Tell us about these addictions."

"They can be any compulsive need, and it's not limited to substance abuse. For example, many parents have a compulsive need to control their children. They insist on unquestioning obedience in order to satisfy their addiction to being in control. Their children grow up as enablers, denying themselves in order to please everyone around them. An enabler often marries an alcoholic, because the alcoholic is addicted to being taken care of, as well as to alcohol. The enabler is addicted to taking care of and pleasing someone, so they make a great co-dependent couple, both cooperating with each other's addictions. When we release our addictions, we transform our lives. Then we can choose to be in a healthy, partnership relationship, in which we are interdependent with our partner, rather than co-dependent."

"You have had some powerful teachers, Sierra."

"That's true. We attract the people into our lives who are the right teachers for us. I have learned that I'm a vehicle to help people heal themselves. Healing does not come from me, rather it comes through me. There are so many ways to heal, subtle ways — for example, creating a safe place in which someone can open up, let their true self come through. So when I counsel, I listen without judgment. That in itself is a form of healing."

"How did you know this was the right path for you?"

"For many years of my life, I prayed to know what I was supposed to do. Then I realized that it was very obvious and comfortable for me to be involved in the area of healing. I knew in my heart that I was on the right path because of the peace I felt — not a peace outside me, but a peace from within and from a spiritual relationship that guides me."

"How do you recommend that people find their higher purpose in life?"

"I believe that when we have a strong intention to find our path, we will find it. We need to trust our intuition, our hearts. When a path feels right, accept it — go for it. Don't hesitate, even if it means changing your life. That's what transformation is all about."

"How can people get in touch with their intuition?"

"Take time to examine a spider web, a flower, or lie on a rock and feel its inspirations flow into you because you created space for it. Hug a tree and feel it hugging you back. Some religions think a close connection with Mother Earth is evil or threatening to their belief system. Nothing is farther from the truth. When we feel the spirit in all living things, how can we deny the presence of Divine Spirit? I believe life is a wonder, an incredible gift. As we return to harmony with the Earth, we will cherish all life more deeply. Then we will take better care of ourselves, our loved ones, and Gaia, our living Earth home."

"Thank you, Sierra. You reinforce the truth that we are all one — all Earthly life is a part of the living,

breathing organism, the Living Spaceship Earth."

Just then a young boy, with long blond hair, dressed in white, approached Maya. He offered her a bouquet of rainbow-colored flowers, with heart-shaped leaves. "These are for you, Maya."

"Thank you. What is your name?"

"Carlos."

Maya experienced pure Galactic love, as she met his gaze. It was Carlos in the form of a young child. "It is time, Maya," he whispered. "All is in readiness."

"Yes, I am ready, Carlos."

Maya watched him disappear behind the stage curtains. She looked at the guests and the audience and began to speak.

"Transformation represents far more than change. It represents a breakthrough to new understanding, heightened awareness, and acceptance of our true selves.

"In order to access your power to transform your life, close your eyes, and take a few moments to breathe deeply, releasing all tension. Now come with me for a walk through a beautiful rainforest. Enjoy the coolness of the air, the fragrance of the jungle flowers, and the feeling of total peace and harmony. Begin walking down the path, and notice an opening in the trees ahead of you. As you reach the trees, the branches part to reveal a gateway to a different dimension of space and time.

"Move through the gateway, knowing that you are perfectly safe and that you are moving toward your unlimited potential. The path takes you to a river, glowing with a mysterious light. Remove your shoes, and experience the soft grass and the warm sand caressing your feet. As you approach the shore, notice that this is no ordinary river. The sparkling, clear water is dancing with the light of millions of precious gemstones and crystals — rose quartz, blue topaz, turquoise, amethysts, emeralds, rubies, sapphires, opals — welcome to Jewel River.

"Now step into its refreshing coolness, letting your-self flow gently with the current. As the jewels brush against your body, sense their radiant colors filling you with awareness of your inner beauty and perfection. Cradle these healing gems in your mind, because they represent the opportunities awaiting you, opportunities to transform your life.... When you are ready, return to the present space and time with the power to achieve a breakthrough to new understanding and heightened awareness, as you use your completed Owner's Manual for your brain.

"Thank you to our guests this evening, Leo, Connie, and Sierra. It has been an honor to serve as your guide for 'High Performance Adventure.' This is Maya Cristal reminding you to use your power of choice to bring about personal and planetary transformation. Good night!"

Announcer: "You may obtain a written transcript of this program and a corresponding Transformation Brainware package by calling the number appearing on your television screen."

Chapter 28

The Path of the Heart

Galactic Agent Josh welcomed Maya with the Mayatan greeting. She nodded knowingly, as she mirrored his salutation.

"You have remembered, my teacher," he communicated telepathically.

"Yes, Josh, for some time. The memories returned slowly, at first, and very rapidly during my experience with T.H.E.M. This afternoon as I was running among the sacred rock formations near my Earth home, I felt my legs getting stronger and stronger with each stride, until I began to sense that I was flying over the ground. Then in an instant, I was within the sacred cave for Galactic Learnings. It was there that I confirmed Rich's identity as a Galactic Agent, and I received a complete energy transmission for the return to Mayata."

"You are aware, then, that all is in readiness for the return home."

"Yes, dear friend. I am aware of all the secrets of the Galaxies. I recognize that for the present, my mission on the Earth plane is complete. And I also have deciphered my encodings from the Galactic energy transmission and know that Carlos has developed a way for us to send macro-laser transmissions from Mayata to the Earthlings."

"Maya, Galactic Agent Rich will now prepare you for your journey."

The presence of an advanced soul entered her awareness, greeting her with joy. "I will miss you, Maya, more than I like to admit. It was a great honor to be a part of this mission."

"You were the best disguised Galactic Agent, Producer Land."

Rich smiled, and for a moment he and Maya held each other in a warm embrace. "Until you fully remembered your powers, my Galactic encodings and the integrity of this mission would not allow me to reach out to you in this way, although I have often dreamed of holding you. Maybe on the next mission we will have more time together. I look forward to your transmissions, and ultimately to your return on future missions. But now, we must disengage your remaining Earthling encodings."

Maya began breathing deeply, entering an altered state of consciousness. "Focus on each breath," directed Rich, "releasing all human programming, until you experience yourself as pure thought.... That's it. Now you're there. Congratulations on a flawless mission."

"Thank you, Rich. It has been a passionate adventure!"

Epilogue

And Gaia Smiled

Maya gazed at the opening in the clouds, blue-white light — starry cosmos leading me home. I see it now, the crystal starship, awaiting my arrival, hovering over the treetops. Iridescent, blue-violet ship, powered by crystalline energy, lights flashing the Mayatan greeting. I am transported into the translucent ship, as it hovers above me, and I walk through the veil that separates Earth-time from the time beyond time.

One brief pause to again view Chichen Itza. It is the Solstice, the moment of transformation into my next reality. Pyramid of Past and Future Reality, you have served me well. Transporting now on my five harmonic tones, tones of perfection, carrying me on a wave of blue, green, rose, violet, and golden light.

Fluid connections to the Universe, accessing all knowledge — all Power, Love, Healing, Wisdom, and Understanding.

Galactic self, I sink into my full awareness, blending with the breath of life. Faster now the ship revolves around my friends, the Earthlings, and their Living Spaceship Earth. My love and energy surround you in warm, golden light.

△ △ △

In the new beginning, the Earthlings chose the path of the heart. As they used their Owner's Manuals to bring about personal and planetary transformation, the Living Spaceship Earth returned to harmony and ecological balance.

AND GAIA SMILED.

THE BEGINNING ...

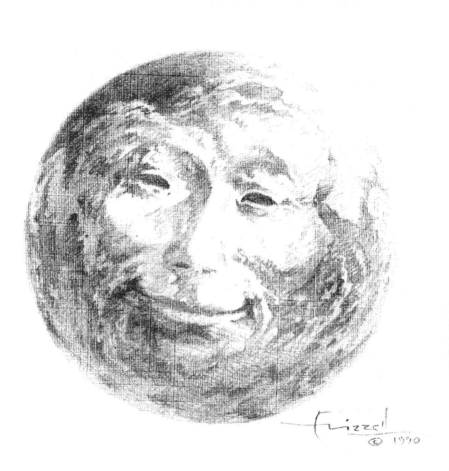

AND

GAIA

SMILED

Owner's Manual Quotes

Chapter 4: Love your fear, and it will release you.

Chapter 6: I used to feel sorry for myself. Then I got to figurin' out who had been makin' all those dumb choices in my life, and it was me.

We are always responsible for our actions.

Only 7 percent of the communications process is the spoken word. The other 93 percent consists of all the unconscious signals that we are constantly sending and receiving.

Chapter 7: Do not attempt to understand me. Concentrate on understanding yourself.

Don't worry about what they say — just keep them talking!

Chapter 8: It is up to you to choose the thoughts that remain in your mind.

I see the world from the eagle's point of view.

Healing deals with the cause of our illness. Curing just deals with the symptoms.

As long as you hold hatred and bitterness in your heart, you will not heal emotional wounds.

Chapter 10: Children and adults fear the unknown much more than the known.

Tolerance is very important. Any time we point a finger at anyone, we are pointing three fingers at ourselves.

Our judgment, blame, intolerance, hatred — all of these harm us much more than the other person.

We don't need to go around the world to find truth. It is right here, within us.

We draw the people and the events in our lives to us because we need to learn something from them.

All diseases are caused by what we think and how we react to life. Both good and evil are self-imposed.

If we love others and give to them, expecting them to give to us in return, then that is not love — that is commerce.

Love plus understanding equals happiness. Hatred plus intolerance equals disaster.

Whenever any book claims to have all the answers, then those who believe totally in that theory are not free, but slaves to their book.

To know the known is to keep the unknown hidden.

There are many paths to truth.

Whenever we judge another, we are only hurting ourselves.

Much more important than what we say is who we are and what actions we take.

Sight may cause some to not see the obvious.

Trust is a spiritual state of mind.

It's vital to our survival that we reconnect with our Earth home through ceremony and ritual.

We need to be more balanced — not always in our analytical minds.

A frightened person lives in a frightening world — a trusting person lives in a trusting world.

Chapter 11: Life as you have ordered it has arrived.

Remember your nobility. Nothing — no one can keep you in bondage without your permission.

It is my right to choose trust over fear, love over apathy, healing over pain.

Your wisdom and understanding are reflected in the choices that you have made.

Chapter 12: We bring about what we think about.

There is no deeper affirmation of who we really are than to say, 'I am.' Action follows this statement quickly.

It is a proven fact that affirmations work. It's simply a matter of which affirmations we use — positive or dysfunctional.

Affirmation statements create a blueprint for success.

We can make the choice to create our own reality.

We affirm what we want, and then we go to work to create it.

We draw to us whatever we expect — whatever we believe we deserve.

When individuals are concerned about losing their freedom, they are not free.

Teach love, not fear. When we release fear, we can fill our lives with love.

Love is natural. Fear must always be programmed.

Chapter 13: Attitude alone does not bring about change.

Our Living Spaceship Earth must return to balance or die a miserable death, choking on her own waste.

Chapter 14: The unknown becomes known when you walk with God.

I would rather live half a life fully than a full life halfway.

Is it too simple an answer to replace fear with love? War with peace? Ecodisaster with ecobalance?

Finding your dream and living it is what life is all about.

Passion is living at your edges and giving 100 percent. To do less is treason against yourself.

Life is either a passionate adventure or it is nothing!

Chapter 15: To understand and not act is not to understand.

Chapter 16: You don't have to swallow the bad peanuts.

Chapter 18: When faced with a mountain, I find a way to get over the top or tunnel through. I never quit!

Don't tell me can't. Can't is not in my vocabulary.

Never, never, never accept a life that doesn't fit.

It is much easier to change your fear of success than to accept less than your potential.

Chapter 20: It is sad that we consider pregnancy an illness and delivery a medical emergency!

Chapter 21: Truth that is organized will cause utter destruction.

Chapter 22: Defining anything tends to restrict it.

Ideas are like children. They must be nurtured and allowed to grow and mature.

The death of creativity is over-organization and obedience to rules and regulations.

Our learning experiences are based on the premise of Plato — that all wisdom is remembering.

When we give children war toys, we are teaching a war mentality.

There are no learning disabled children, only learning disabled teaching methods.

Dreams give birth to reality.

Within each of us there is a magical, childlike, creative self who is waiting to be welcomed back into our lives.

Chapter 23: It just doesn't make sense to be destroying our natural resources for the sake of a self-centered, unhealthy lifestyle.

Chapter 24: Change has to start with each individual making a difference!

As we put aside our nationalism and work together

with other countries, we will be able to bring about a peace and a healing of the Earth.

Choose to exercise your personal power by taking action to return the Earth to balance and harmony.

Chapter 26: To encapsulate TRUTH into religious dogma, no matter how pure the intent, would be repeating the mistakes of the past.

Until you learn to be in partnership with your feminine and masculine energy, then you are only half a person.

Pure spirit brought to Earth has always been misunderstood — condemned as the Devil by some — worshiped by others. Pure spirit simply is.

Chapter 27: Your perception equals your reality.

It's masculine energy — the masculine energy in both men and women that has been out of balance for thousands of years.

Change is inevitable — growth is optional.

Every moment is special.

There are no victims — only volunteers.

We attract the people into our lives who are the right teachers for us.

Life is a series of choices, and we have to be willing to take responsibility for the consequences of those choices.

The macho man is a dinosaur.

My greatest lesson has been to live in the moment, to accept myself and everything around me as perfect in each moment.

The ways of native peoples have been to live in harmony and balance, adapting themselves to Mother Earth.

It is imperative that we heal ourselves before we can heal the planet.

We are not in this world to live up to others' expectations.

Partnership is transforming our family systems, the way we raise and educate our children, our relationships, our workplace, our government, and our attitude and actions toward our planet.

When we have a strong intention to find our path, we will find it. We need to trust our intuition, our hearts. When a path feels right, accept it.

Transformation represents a breakthrough to new understanding, heightened awareness, and acceptance of our true selves.

Use your power of choice to bring about personal and planetary transformation.

Epilogue: In the new beginning, the Earthlings chose the path of the heart.

Δ Δ Δ

Typesetting by PineCastle™ Type & Graphics, Ltd.

Charles Frizzell

ARTIST, VISIONARY, ENVIRONMENTALIST

The painting on the cover of *Do You Have an Owner's Manual for Your Brain?* reflects the visionary genius of Frizzell art. Like all Frizzell paintings, it is more than paint and canvas — it is love, beauty, and mystical perfection. His paintings mirror his quiet brilliance and tireless attention to minute detail.

Charles works in a partnership relationship with his wife, Shawn, whose intuitive senses and spiritual energy have guided him into a visionary art that inspires and nourishes the soul — stimulating individuals to find peace and balance within, realizing their relation with the whole of life.

The Frizzells are actively involved in the movement to return the Earth to ecobalance through Charles' paintings and Shawn's active role in their mountain community of Victor, Colorado. She is an herbalist, counselor, healer, and environmental activist.

America and the world are rapidly awakening to Frizzell masterpieces that are available in limited edition prints, art posters, originals, and greeting cards.

For information on their extraordinary art write to:

Frizzell Studios
P.O. Box 495
Victor, CO 80860
or call (719) 689-2232

To: Action Press, P.O. Box 6250, Colorado Springs, CO 80934
719-577-9577

Please send me the following:	Price	Qty.	Total
Do You Have an Owner's Manual for Your Brain? by Marina Raye	$12.95		
ABZ's of High Performance by Chuck Sheppard	9.95		
Maya, The Starchild (book cover art) Poster by Charles Frizzell (24 x 18 color)	19.95		

Subtotal _____

Colorado Residents: Add 6.5% sales tax _____
Shipping: Add $2.05 for first item ordered,
$1 each additional item _____

(U.S. Funds only) **TOTAL** _____

SHIP TO: Name _____

Street or P.O. Box _____

City _____ State _____ Zip _____
PAYMENT: ❑ Check ❑ Visa ❑ MasterCard
Card # _____ Exp. Date _____

_____   _____
Print Cardholder's Name   Cardholder's Signature

• DEALER INQUIRIES WELCOME •

Coming soon from Action Press

Brainware™ — The Workbook
for *Do You Have an Owner's Manual for Your Brain?*
by Marina Raye

For information on Marina Raye's *Owner's Manual* Workshops,
Dreammaker Seminars, and speaking engagements, contact:
Action Press, P.O. Box 6250, Colorado Springs, CO 80934

719-577-9577